Praise for **The Motivation Mindset Workbook**

"This indispensable resource gives teens the tools to discover what motivates them (and what doesn't), what their goals are, and the action steps they can take to move toward those goals. The exercises are quick and easy and offer a range of options for kids to choose the best fit. Most important, the book helps teens build self-awareness and a sense of control over the direction of their lives. Highly recommended!"

—**Richard Guare, PhD, BCBA-D, author of**
Smart but Scattered

"I appreciate the way that kids are invited to take ownership of their own priorities at every step. I'm very grateful to have this wonderful book in my parenting toolkit!"

—**Clare B., Pittsburgh**

"Drs. Braaten and Bush go beyond explaining *why* kids struggle with motivation—they give us concrete, age-appropriate ways to explore the *how* of helping kids connect with what matters to them. The self-reflective activities invite teens and tweens to better understand their own strengths, needs, and motivators—and will help parents and educators make discoveries about themselves, too. This book offers a rare and welcome blend of insight, empathy, and real-world application."

—**Amanda Morin, educational consultant**
and author of *Adulting Made Easy*

"As the mother of two bright and curious kids, it's always frustrating when they don't seem to want to do anything. This book has a ton of suggestions to help all of us work through what's making things difficult. I really appreciate that there are exercises and conversation ideas that will speak to both of my children, who have very different personalities. Anything that increases my options for helping my kids get more motivated is great!"

—**Krista L., Boston**

"The authors approach motivation from different perspectives—all research based—and provide practical activities for a range of ages. I appreciate the emphasis on encouraging teens and tweens to identify their own interests, strengths, and values, rather than solely trying to meet others' expectations. I recommend this book for parents, caregivers, and any young person who could use help overcoming barriers to success."

—Hilary Adams, PhD, Clinical Director,
Therapy Lab Kids

The Motivation Mindset Workbook

Also Available

The
Motivation
Mindset
WORKBOOK

Helping Teens and Tweens
Discover What They Love to Do

Ellen Braaten, PhD
Hillary Bush, PhD

gp

THE GUILFORD PRESS

New York   London

Copyright © 2026 The Guilford Press
A Division of Guilford Publications, Inc.
www.guilford.com

Printed in the United States of America

For product and safety concerns within the EU, please contact
GPSR@taylorandfrancis.com, Taylor & Francis Verlag GmbH, Kaufingerstraße 24,
80331 München, Germany.

Last digit is print number: 9   8   7   6   5   4   3   2   1

This publication is intended to provide helpful and informative material. It is not
intended to diagnose, treat, cure, or prevent any health problem or condition, nor is
it intended to replace the advice of a health professional. No action should be taken
based solely on the contents of this book. Always consult your physician or qualified
health care professional on any matters regarding your health and before adopting
any suggestions in this book or drawing inferences from it.

    The authors and publisher specifically disclaim all responsibility for any liability,
loss, or risk, personal or otherwise, which is incurred as a consequence, directly or
indirectly, from the use or application of any contents of this book.

    Any and all product names referenced within this book are the trademarks of
their respective owners. Always read all information provided by the manufacturers'
product labels before using their products. The authors and publisher are not
responsible for claims made by manufacturers.

Library of Congress Cataloging-in-Publication Data is available from the publisher.

ISBN 978-1-4625-5558-1 (paperback) — ISBN 978-1-4625-5926-8 (hardcover)

With gratitude to the families and students
who have inspired my work

—E. B.

For Devon, Tipton, and Theodore,
the loves of my life

—H. B.

Contents

Acknowledgments

We are infinitely grateful for the wisdom and insight of our editors, Kitty Moore and Chris Benton. Thank you for believing in this project and for your spot-on guidance throughout every step of the process.

We gratefully acknowledge Megan Murray and her expert management of our clinical work. Thank you for everything you do to keep our professional lives running smoothly!

The process of writing this workbook continually reminded us that physical health is health and that mental health is health too. We are grateful for all the professionals who helped us care for ourselves as we embarked on this project.

Our gratitude for our patients is endless. Thank you for entrusting us with your care and for inviting us into your lives. Your determination, strength, creativity, and humor are woven throughout the activities in this workbook.

From the bottom of our hearts, we thank our dear friends and family. You motivate us and keep us moving forward every day.

* * *

The VIA Institute on Character has generously given permission to adapt material from M. Jermann and R. E. McGrath (2022), *Revision of the VIA Inventory of Strengths for Youth: 1. Item Development, Selection, and Initial Validation*, used in the worksheet "Field Trip! . . . to the VIA Institute on Character" on pages 33–35.

Introduction

For Parents and Professionals

There are few things more frustrating than being the parent, teacher, or therapist of an unmotivated child. Unmotivated kids don't fit into a single category; they're not just depressed, or anxious, or disorganized, or learning disabled, or addicted to video games—just to name a few of the behaviors unmotivated kids might display. Some unmotivated kids have a lot of these behaviors, and others have almost none. But they all share one trait: *they don't seem to care a whole lot about much of anything.* Parents, other caregivers, and teachers of these kids tend to feel hopeless, helpless, and worried about the child's future prospects. Getting them back on track can feel like an impossible task.

In 2023, one of us (Ellen) wrote a book about these kids called *Bright Kids Who Couldn't Care Less.* The book explored the issue of kids who didn't care from many different vantage points, from understanding a child's individual differences to reflecting on what might have caused a child to lose interest. Parents were encouraged to analyze their own expectations and reflect on their child's unique qualities and were taught how to set goals. But many parents, teachers, and clinicians wanted more practical, experiential activities—they wanted things they could *do,* and in that spirit this book was born.

Chapter 1 of this book—"What's the Point?"—identifies the importance of motivation and the problems that occur without it. The following aspects of not caring, and more, are explored:

- **What is motivation?**

- **What does motivation look like in the child in your life? Is a certain part of motivation particularly hard for the child? Getting started? Staying motivated? A lack of interest?**

- **What are the sorts of things motivated people tend to believe? Are they things that jibe with how you see yourself?**

Chapter 2—"Who Am I?"—can help you identify a child's strengths. Kids who have lost motivation have often lost a sense of what they're good at. Sometimes there's a mismatch between what the adults in their life think they're good at and what they're actually capable of doing. Maybe a lot of attention has been paid to the things a child is *not* doing. This chapter helps children think about themselves in new ways. If they're having trouble identifying their strengths, the activities in this chapter will help. Using the worksheets will help them articulate who they are—and who they are *not*.

Chapter 3 poses the question "What Makes Me Happy?" because the answer to this question is an essential component in staying motivated. Unmotivated kids live in a world where nearly everything seems unappealing. The activities in this chapter help them focus on what does, or at least *could,* make them happy, while Chapter 4 provides activities that answer the question "How Can I Get More of What Makes Me Happy?" Chapter 5, "Pulling It All Together," helps kids, well, pull it all together, using the knowledge gained in the preceding chapters, to make appropriate goals, revise goals, and obtain insight into how others can help them achieve their goals.

Finally, motivation doesn't happen in isolation from the rest of daily life. Sleep, anxiety, screen time, stress, and exercise all can interfere with—or enhance—motivation. Chapter 6, "A Few Other Things That Can Get in the Way of Motivation," provides go-to examples of how to address these important areas. At the back of the book you'll find Resources that offer our favorite recommendations for further reading and support.

How to Use This Workbook

We devised this workbook to be used in a variety of ways. Kids who lack motivation are not typically moved to pick up a workbook and start writing. That's why most of these activities are short and meant to be shared with the adults in the child's life. It's also why we've included some quotations about other kids' experiences, to inspire children's imagination as well as affirm how common it is to feel unmotivated. These quotes are representative of what we've heard from children and teenagers over the years but are fictional. These worksheets are for children and adolescents, from approximately ages 8 to 16, but some can be used with younger children, and some topics are even appropriate for adults.

Clinicians and educators may lead individuals or groups of children or teenagers to work on concepts and share what they've discovered. But whether you're a parent working with your own individual child or leading a group, the children and teens who work with you through this book will learn about what gives them pleasure, begin to understand the basic concepts of motivation, discover more about their strengths and weaknesses, and become better prepared to integrate these ideas into a way to help them feel and act more motivated. What's more, you'll feel less helpless, strengthen the bond you have with your child or students, teach them important concepts, and help them thrive and become more fully themselves. You might even find yourself learning something more about yourself. Although the activities in the book are fairly self-explanatory, they are meant to complement, not to substitute for, the content in *Bright Kids Who Couldn't Care Less (BKWCCL)*. The activities in this book will be more meaningful if you're already familiar with the concepts explored in *BKWCCL*.

These worksheets don't need to be done sequentially. Not every child will benefit from doing every activity, but most kids will benefit from some attention to each of the chapters. Pick and choose the activities that seem most appropriate for an individual child's interests and development. That being said, a good place to start is with

Chapter 1, as it helps the child understand the concept of motivation and why it's important. You can use activities from Chapters 2, 3, and 4 simultaneously. Pick one or two activities at a time from each area. The goal is to integrate the answers to these questions into a way to rekindle motivation, explored in Chapter 5. When you run into road-blocks, or you know your child has a problem with sleep, anxiety, or social media (just a few of the topics covered), use the activities in Chapter 6 as a way of gaining more information and skills to help. If that's not enough, you can take a look at the resources we've collected at the back of the book.

Overall, the activities in each chapter ask the participant to *reflect* on the past, *take action* in the present, and/or *set goals* for the future, all in the hope of helping the child develop a more complete sense of self. If you are a parent, you may decide to use this book more as a guide than as a set of activities. If you are a teacher or a therapist, you may choose to use these activities in individual or group settings. Motivation ebbs and flows throughout our lives, and these activities are ones that can be used again and again as children discover new things about themselves.

We know it's scary to look into the future when you've got an unmotivated child in your life. On a daily basis, we hear questions like "Will he ever like anything?" and "Why doesn't she care anymore?" along with statements such as "I'm positive they'll be living with me for the rest of their life." We've written this book to provide hope, tools, and activities to help parents and professionals feel less stuck so that adults and kids can experience a more meaningful, happier life that leaves them feeling motivated for what's ahead. We hope you find it helpful and supportive.

1

What's the Point?

The activities in the following pages answer the questions "What is motivation?" and "How does it affect me?" Motivation is the *why* we do the things we do, and these activities help children and teens become familiar with different kinds of motivation and how each of these fits into their life and personality. Motivation is not a single character trait. It's not something that is "built into" us. It's complicated and affected by our biology, support system, opportunities for rewards, and desire to keep our lives running smoothly. Motivation is different for everyone—and it can change over time and in response to circumstances.

No single theory—and no single worksheet in this chapter—will unlock the secrets of motivation. It's a complicated topic, and thinking about it from many different angles is a good place to start. Use this chapter as a launching pad before tackling the nuts and bolts of motivation in the chapters that follow.

The first few worksheets (pages 7–12) give kids the opportunity to start thinking about motivation as well as where or why they might be stuck. The middle activities (pages 13–17) are a little more educational—giving kids some knowledge about motivation—while asking them to reflect on how each of these theories impacts their own lives. The final worksheet (page 18) presents the concepts that are well covered in the next few chapters, setting the stage to get children and teens thinking about what gives them *pleasure,* what they like to do (*practice),* and what they're naturally good at doing (*aptitude*).

Starting to Get Started

Getting started on an activity or task—whether you feel fully ready to begin or not so ready at all—is an important part of motivation. Many things can make it hard for us to get started. Below are hills with the situations and thoughts that often get in the way of taking the first step. Color in or highlight the ones that feel most true for you. If you have other ideas, a few hills are blank so you can write them in.

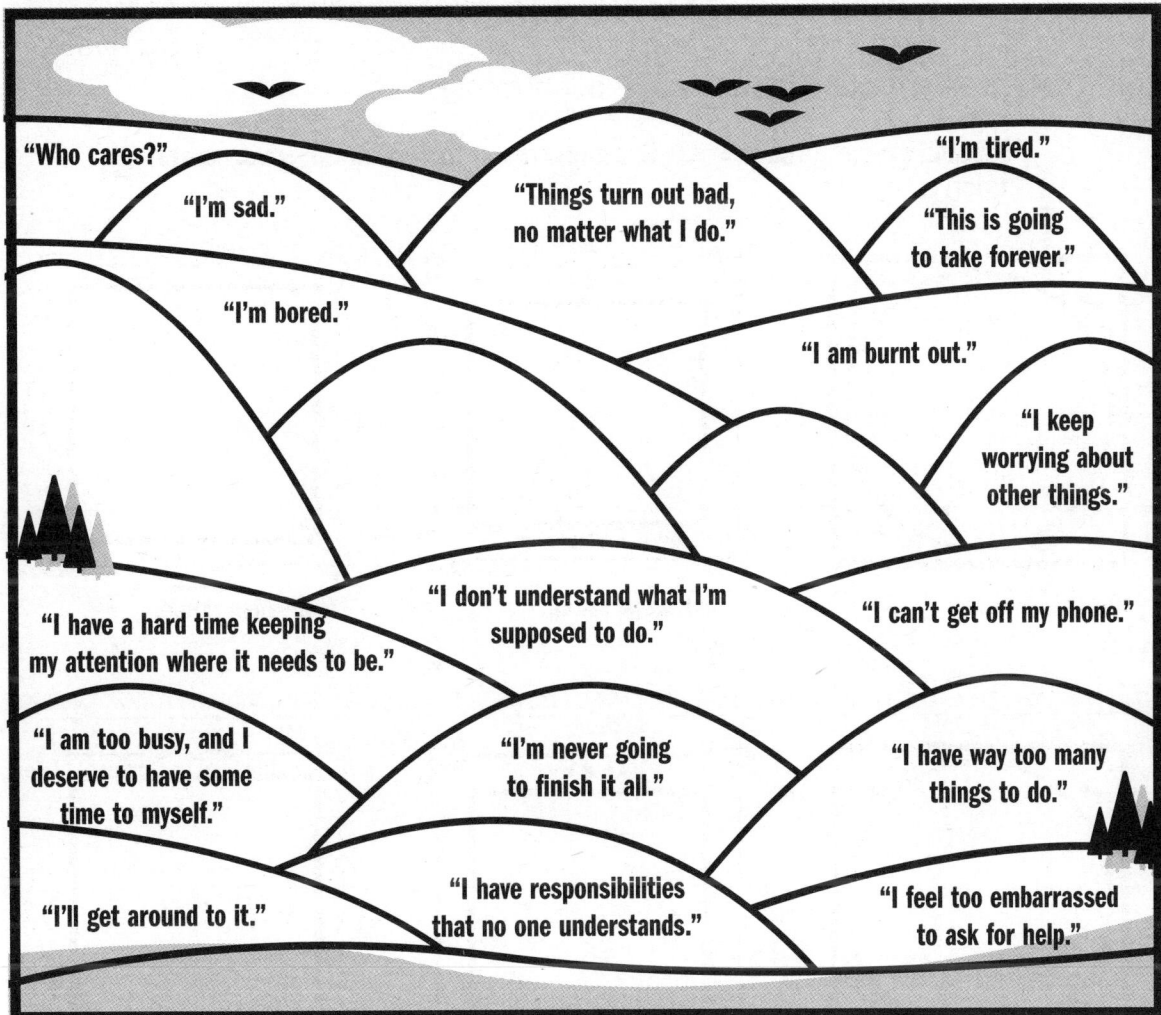

"Who cares?"
"I'm sad."
"I'm tired."
"Things turn out bad, no matter what I do."
"This is going to take forever."
"I'm bored."
"I am burnt out."
"I keep worrying about other things."
"I don't understand what I'm supposed to do."
"I can't get off my phone."
"I have a hard time keeping my attention where it needs to be."
"I am too busy, and I deserve to have some time to myself."
"I'm never going to finish it all."
"I have way too many things to do."
"I'll get around to it."
"I have responsibilities that no one understands."
"I feel too embarrassed to ask for help."

Look at what you've highlighted. *Any ideas about why these get in your way?*

_____

_____

People Who Motivate Me . . . and People Who Don't

You interact with lots of people every day—your mom, dad, friends, teachers, coaches, and grandparents—just to name a few. Interacting with others has a big impact on how motivated you feel—or don't feel. For this activity, think about the people you spend the most time with. You can draw a picture or write their names in the frames below. Give each person a rating from 0 (not at all) to 10 (the highest) to reflect how often or how much they motivate you. Then briefly write why you gave each rating.

> "I would give my nana a 10! She believes in me so much—even when I don't."
> —MILA, AGE 14

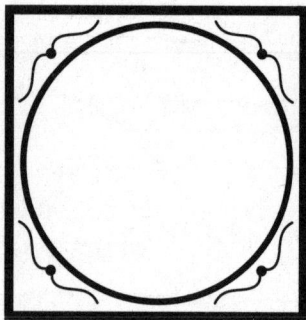

Motivation rating: _____
Why? _____

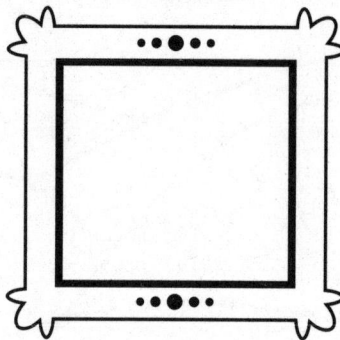

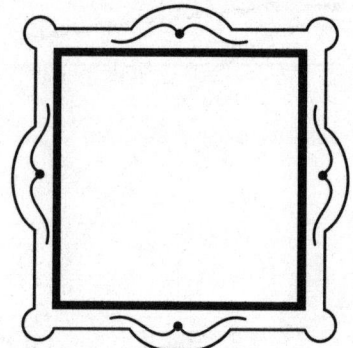

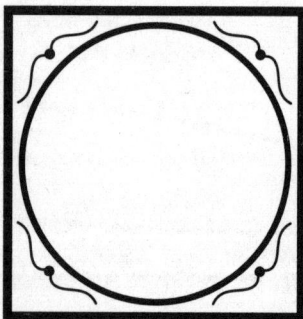

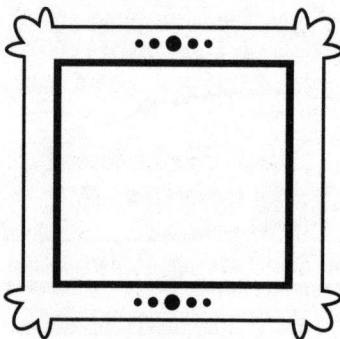

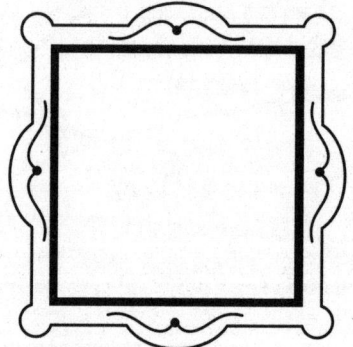

Motivation rating: _____
Why? _____

Motivation rating: _____
Why? _____

Motivation rating: _____
Why? _____

Motivation rating: _____
Why? _____

Motivation rating: _____
Why? _____

Stalling Out

Do you have trouble getting started? Lots of kids do, and it can look different depending on what you've got to do. Knowing where you tend to have trouble is an important first step toward making changes.

In the chart below are some areas where kids commonly have problems with **initiation** (or getting started). As you read, ask yourself: Where do I struggle? What comes easily?

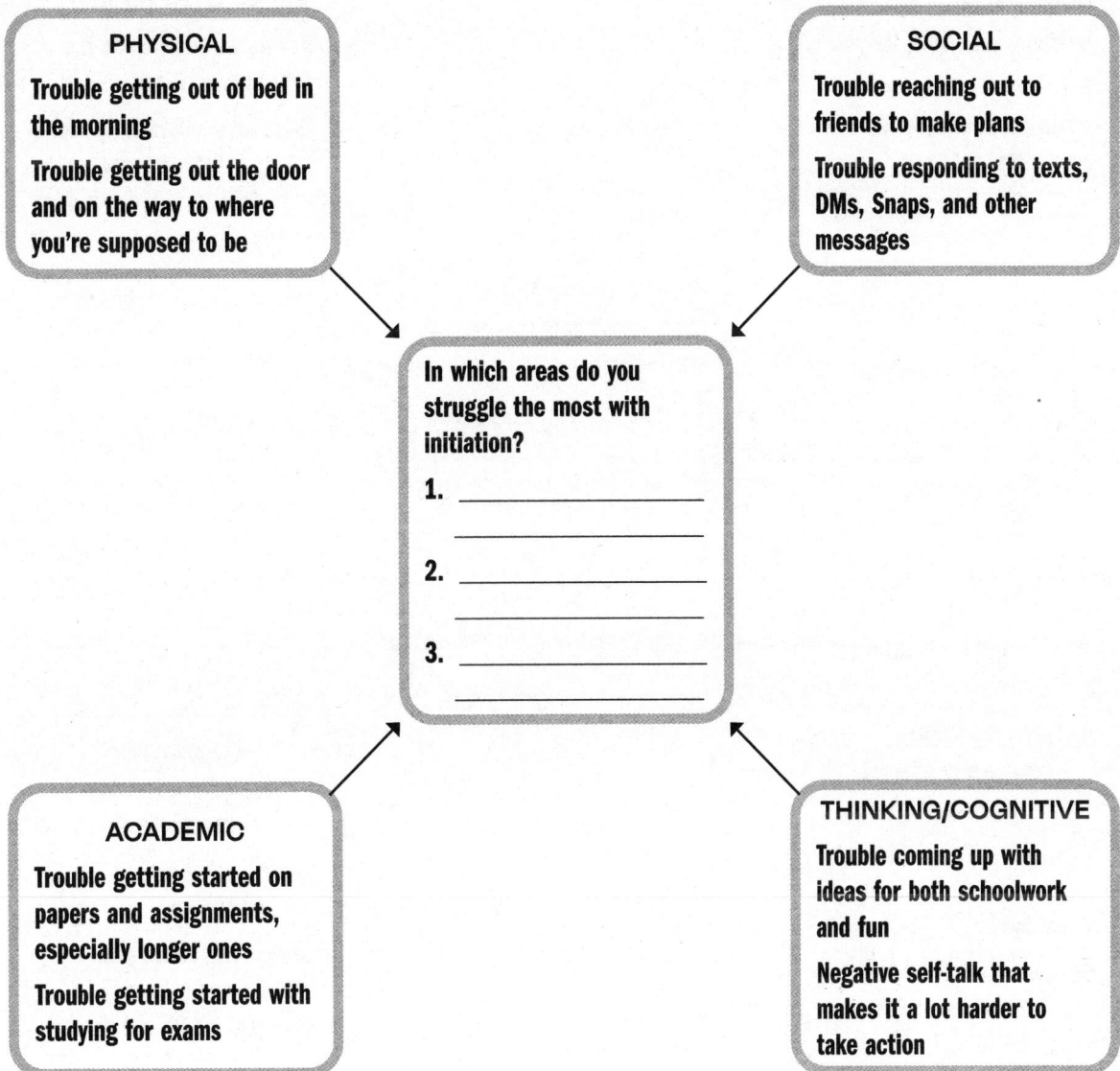

PHYSICAL

Trouble getting out of bed in the morning

Trouble getting out the door and on the way to where you're supposed to be

SOCIAL

Trouble reaching out to friends to make plans

Trouble responding to texts, DMs, Snaps, and other messages

In which areas do you struggle the most with initiation?

1. _____
   _____
2. _____
   _____
3. _____
   _____

ACADEMIC

Trouble getting started on papers and assignments, especially longer ones

Trouble getting started with studying for exams

THINKING/COGNITIVE

Trouble coming up with ideas for both schoolwork and fun

Negative self-talk that makes it a lot harder to take action

For Real Getting Started

As hard as it can be to get started, especially on tasks that we find unpleasant, fortunately there are some ways of getting started (for real). Which ones do you think might be helpful to you?

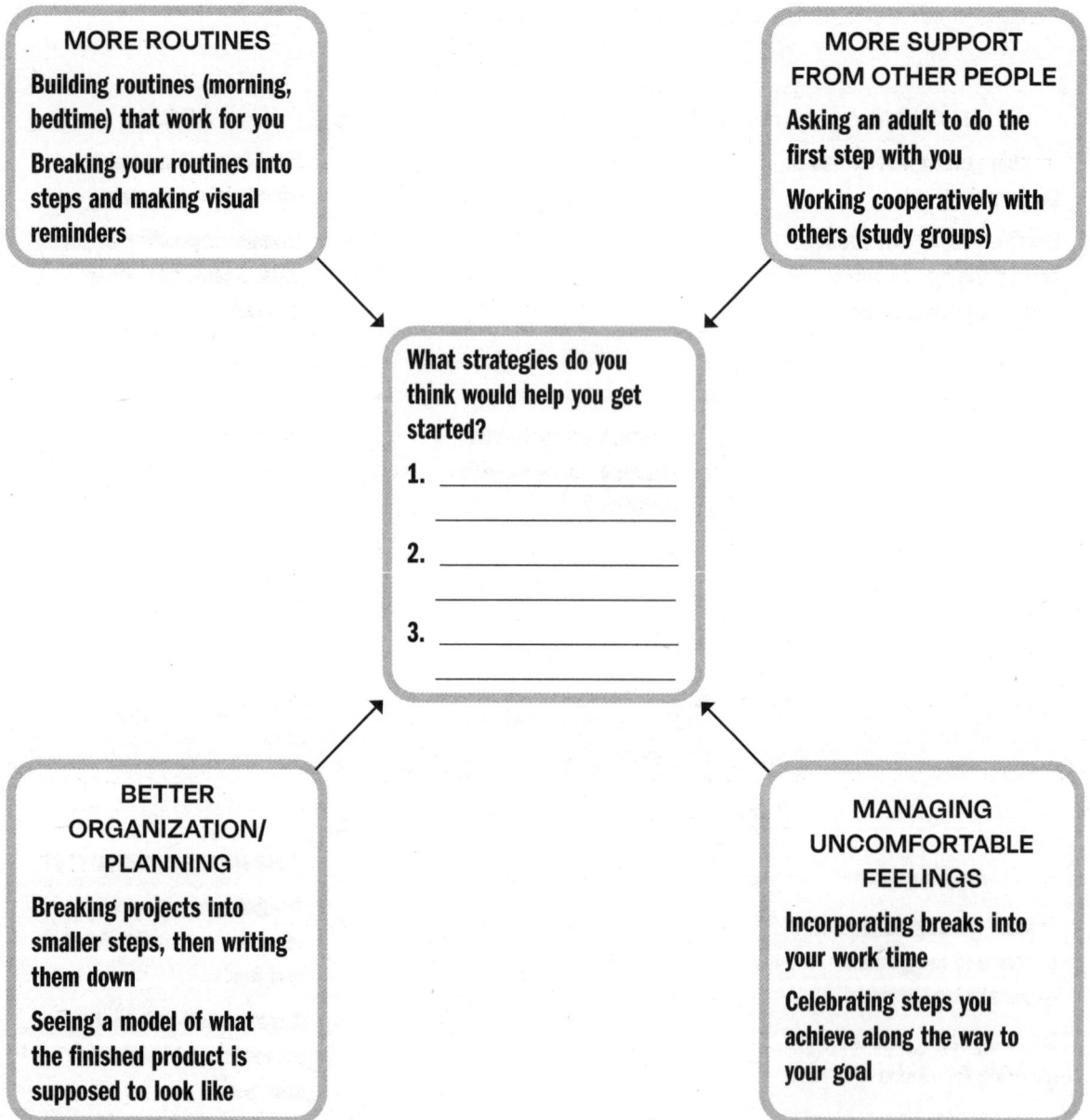

MORE ROUTINES

Building routines (morning, bedtime) that work for you

Breaking your routines into steps and making visual reminders

MORE SUPPORT FROM OTHER PEOPLE

Asking an adult to do the first step with you

Working cooperatively with others (study groups)

What strategies do you think would help you get started?

1. _____
_____
2. _____
_____
3. _____
_____

BETTER ORGANIZATION/ PLANNING

Breaking projects into smaller steps, then writing them down

Seeing a model of what the finished product is supposed to look like

MANAGING UNCOMFORTABLE FEELINGS

Incorporating breaks into your work time

Celebrating steps you achieve along the way to your goal

Where Am I Getting Stuck?

There are three important parts of motivation: **initiation** (getting started on the thing you want to do or are supposed to do), **intensity** (how hard—or not hard—you work on that thing), and **persistence** (how long—or not long—you spend doing that thing, without getting off track or stopping completely). When your initiation, intensity, and persistence are all strong, your motivation looks terrific and you can work hard and get a lot done. However, when one or more of these areas is weak, it can be hard to do the things you want—or even *need*—to do.

As you read the scenarios below, ask yourself **"Where am I getting stuck?"** In the "My Rating" box, insert a **1** for the area that causes you the **most difficulty,** a **2** for the area that causes you the second most difficulty, and a **3** for the area that causes you the third most difficulty.

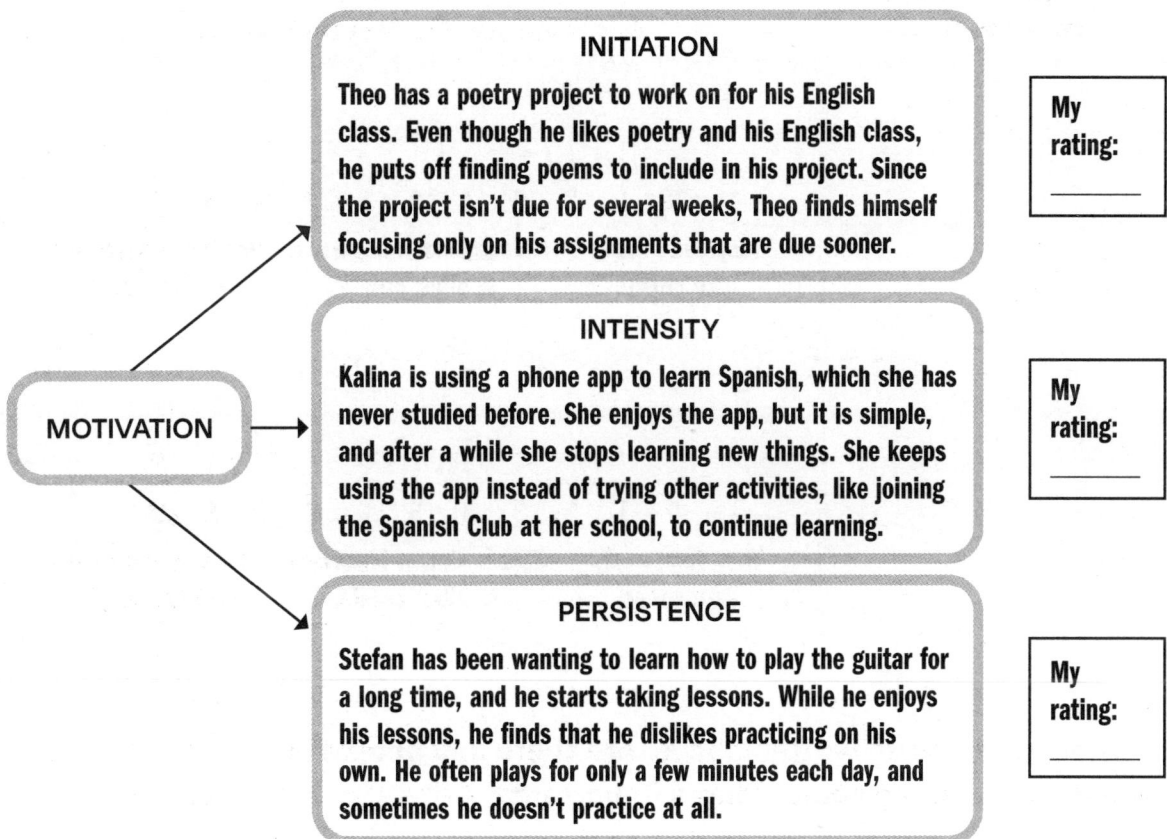

MOTIVATION

INITIATION

Theo has a poetry project to work on for his English class. Even though he likes poetry and his English class, he puts off finding poems to include in his project. Since the project isn't due for several weeks, Theo finds himself focusing only on his assignments that are due sooner.

My rating:

_____

INTENSITY

Kalina is using a phone app to learn Spanish, which she has never studied before. She enjoys the app, but it is simple, and after a while she stops learning new things. She keeps using the app instead of trying other activities, like joining the Spanish Club at her school, to continue learning.

My rating:

_____

PERSISTENCE

Stefan has been wanting to learn how to play the guitar for a long time, and he starts taking lessons. While he enjoys his lessons, he finds that he dislikes practicing on his own. He often plays for only a few minutes each day, and sometimes he doesn't practice at all.

My rating:

_____

What Are the Things I Don't Care About?

Sometimes it can be helpful to name the things you really don't care about. It might even be possible to let some of these things go. And it's good to know the ones you cannot let go. In the chart below, fill in some of the things that you don't care about (even if some people think you should). Next to each one, insert an **X** where you think other people feel about it.

> "My parents keep encouraging me to run for student government. They say I'm a 'natural leader.' I guess it's nice of them to say and think that, but I'm really not interested in student government—and especially not running for office." —SOO, AGE 15

I just don't care about . . .

But other people feel this way . . .

0 1 2 3 4 5 6 7 8 9 10

They don't really care either!   This is kind of important to other people.   It's really important to other people.

0 1 2 3 4 5 6 7 8 9 10

They don't really care either!   This is kind of important to other people.   It's really important to other people.

Look at what you've written above. **Are there any people in particular with whom you disagree about what's important?** Write about it here:

_____

_____

Maslow's Hierarchy of Needs

There are a number of theories that try to explain how motivation works. In the 1940s psychologist Abraham Maslow wrote that people need to meet certain basic needs (like having food, sleep, and warmth) before they can achieve other goals, like friendship and motivation. In other words, it's hard to be motivated if you're hungry or tired. Below is a pyramid that shows Maslow's hierarchy of needs. The needs closer to the bottom are basic needs, while the ones closer to the top are more complex. To achieve at the top, you've got to satisfy the needs at the bottom.

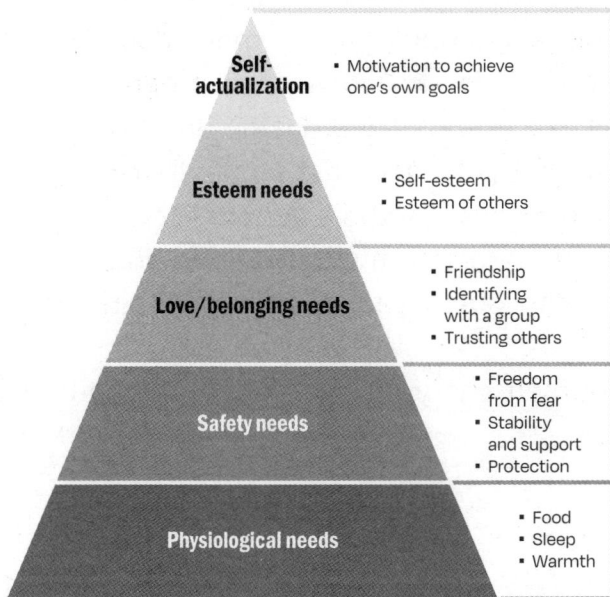

Self-actualization
- Motivation to achieve one's own goals

Esteem needs
- Self-esteem
- Esteem of others

Love/belonging needs
- Friendship
- Identifying with a group
- Trusting others

Safety needs
- Freedom from fear
- Stability and support
- Protection

Physiological needs
- Food
- Sleep
- Warmth

On this graph, insert a star at the level of needs you feel like you are at today.

Do you ever feel like you spend time across different levels of needs? If so, what do you notice, and what does this feel like?

_____

_____

Are there things you feel like you are missing in your life right now that are preventing you from achieving higher-order goals or needs? If so, what are you missing?

_____

_____

Instinct Theory of Motivation

Sometimes we're motivated because of our ***instincts.*** Instincts relate to our biology. Some instincts we're born with. For example, babies *instinctively* turn their heads toward food when their cheeks are touched. They didn't have to learn to do this; they do this *instinctively.* Most animals are motivated by instincts. Birds fly south for the winter. We seek shelter when it's raining and warmth when we're cold. This theory of motivation suggests we all have the same motivations because we all have the same biology. And that biology helps us survive.

This sounds fair enough, right? Still, you can probably see there are problems with this theory. We aren't birds. We don't always make decisions or do things that are in line with our long-term survival. Our preprogrammed motivations are influenced by feelings like jealousy and desire. But biology is something that everyone has, and it accounts—at least somewhat—for why we do the things we do. For example, Jamal and his soccer team were winning a championship game when a thunderstorm occurred. He and his team (and everyone else too) *instinctively* sought shelter from the rain and possible lightning.

Based on what you know about yourself and your own motivation, put an **X** where you fall on the line below.

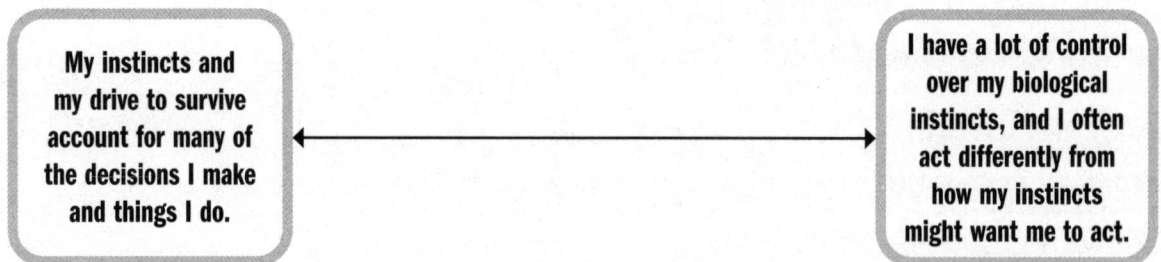

My instincts and my drive to survive account for many of the decisions I make and things I do.	←————————————→	I have a lot of control over my biological instincts, and I often act differently from how my instincts might want me to act.

Incentive Theory of Motivation

The **incentive theory of motivation** explains that we are motivated to do things because someone gives us a reward. For example, adults are motivated to go to work every day because they want to receive a paycheck. Kids and teens are often motivated by getting good grades (if they study for a test), getting positive attention (if they show good behavior), and getting an allowance (if they do chores around the house). We talk a lot more about incentives, including how they can help and how they can hurt, in the coming chapters of this workbook. Incentives can vary a lot from person to person. Something that is super motivating for one person (like going to see a professional basketball game) might feel like punishment for someone else! For example, Kathy wasn't a strong reader, but she was motivated to read books over the summer because she'd get a $50 gift card, while Brad was motivated to read books over the summer because he just loved to read books.

Based on what you know about yourself and your own motivation, put an **X** where you fall on the line below:

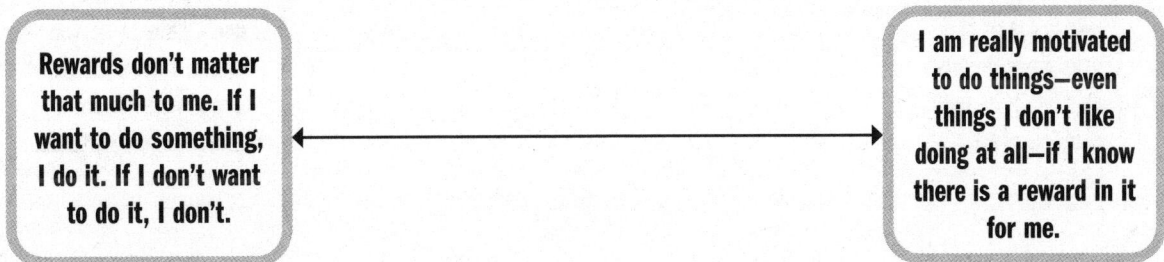

Rewards don't matter that much to me. If I want to do something, I do it. If I don't want to do it, I don't.

←——————————————→

I am really motivated to do things—even things I don't like doing at all—if I know there is a reward in it for me.

Drive Theory of Motivation

Sometimes our motivation is affected by our need to reduce feelings of tension and anxiety. That's the idea behind the **drive theory of motivation.** For example, we are motivated to eat something when we feel hungry, because hunger is an uncomfortable feeling. A student who knows their teacher will be angry or disappointed if homework isn't done might be motivated to complete the assignment. Or a student might be motivated *not* to complete a homework assignment because they are afraid they will not do a good job, and the tension and embarrassment of turning in a poor assignment and looking "stupid" is worse than the tension and embarrassment of an angry teacher. So the drive theory of motivation helps explain why people may show very different behaviors in the same situation—it all comes down to drive.

Based on what you know about yourself and your own motivation, put an **X** where you fall on the line below:

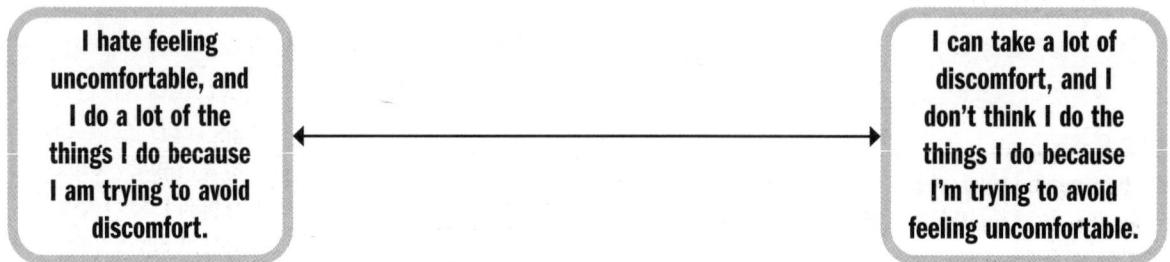

I hate feeling uncomfortable, and I do a lot of the things I do because I am trying to avoid discomfort.	⟷	I can take a lot of discomfort, and I don't think I do the things I do because I'm trying to avoid feeling uncomfortable.

Arousal Theory of Motivation

The **arousal theory of motivation** is all about staying in a state of balance. Arousal, in this case, is about our desire not to be too out of control or too "on edge," but also not to be too bored either. We tend to feel best in the middle. This theory of motivation says that we do things to keep us "right in the middle." For example, if we're too stressed, we might "check out" by playing video games or scrolling through TikTok. When we're bored, we might be apt to watch an exciting TV show or maybe even do something physical that revs us up, like skateboarding.

Based on what you know about yourself and your own motivation, put an **X** where you fall on the line below:

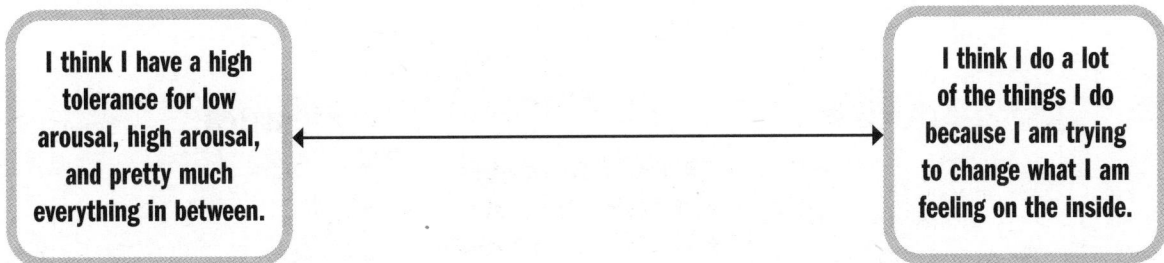

I think I have a high tolerance for low arousal, high arousal, and pretty much everything in between.	←——————————→	I think I do a lot of the things I do because I am trying to change what I am feeling on the inside.

Where Is My Motivation Right Now?

In the following chapters, we think a lot about **aptitude** (Who Am I?), **pleasure** (What Makes Me Happy?), and **practice** (How Can I Get More of What Makes Me Happy?) The overlap of these three areas—aptitude, pleasure, and practice—is where great motivation comes from. The activities in this workbook help you learn more about yourself and what aptitude, pleasure, and practice look like for you. But even before we get into those, you might already have ideas about the activities where your aptitude, pleasure, and practice come together and where you already have a lot of motivation. If you can identify any activities like these (although it's completely OK if you cannot), write them on the lines below:

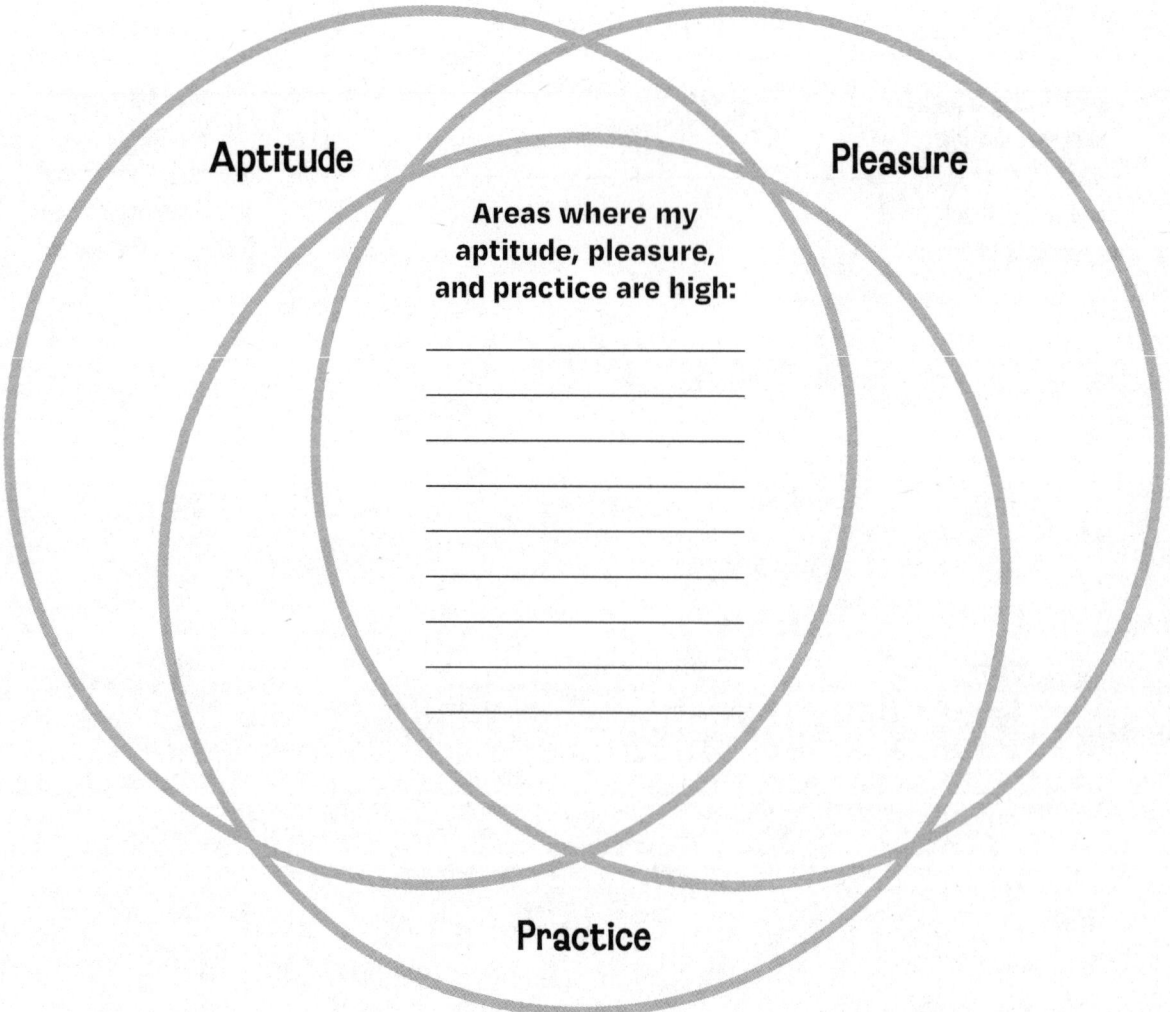

Aptitude   **Pleasure**

Areas where my aptitude, pleasure, and practice are high:

_____
_____
_____
_____
_____
_____
_____
_____

Practice

2

Who Am I?

Chapter 2 gives you a chance to take a deep dive into understanding aptitudes and strengths. The word *aptitude* is often used interchangeably with *ability* or *intellect,* but we like to think of aptitude as *potential* or *innate capabilities*. When adults try to figure out why children don't care about much of anything, they first need to figure out how capable a child is of doing things. Unmotivated kids have often lost the ability to identify their strengths, and without that it's easy to be pulled into negative thinking, setting up a cycle that decreases motivation. Focusing on strengths is important because knowing your areas of competence is associated with decreased stress and positive emotions. Identifying (or, in many cases, reidentifying) their strengths can take some effort for children who have been feeling apathetic for quite some time. It might take a lot of reflection and looking beyond the obvious areas, such as academics and sports, to things like character, leadership qualities, empathy, and social skills. This chapter is filled with activities that help kids answer the questions "Who am I?" and "Who do I want to become?"

The first group of activities (pages 21–30) begins by asking kids to reflect on who they are: Where are they happiest? What makes them sad? Who do they admire? How do they imagine the future? The middle section (pages 31–36) gives kids the opportunity to get some real data on their personality traits and characteristics, using free online, well-researched resources. They can use the information gained from these activities to reflect on their own personality, as well as the personalities of those in the family, since motivation is sometimes a family issue (such as a poor match between personalities and goals within the family system). These worksheets are followed by activities that help children learn more about their character strengths and personality styles (pages 37–48). Finally, the chapter ends with ways to help children apply what they've learned about themselves to increase motivation and purpose in their lives (page 49).

Not all of these activities need to be completed. As you are deciding what activities might be helpful, keep in mind that the purpose of this chapter is self-knowledge. Children should complete enough of these worksheets so they can give reasonable answers to these questions:

- **"Who am I as a person?"**

- **"What are my strengths?"**

- **"What are clearly not my strengths?"**

- **"How do my strengths match the strengths and personalities of other people, especially the adults, in my life?"**

- **"Who is the person I'd like to become?"**

Here I Am

Think about who you are at this moment in time. What do you think about? What do you like to do? What do you NOT like to do? In the frame below, make a self-portrait. How you do this is completely up to you—it can include pictures, sketches, cartoons, words about you, or anything else.

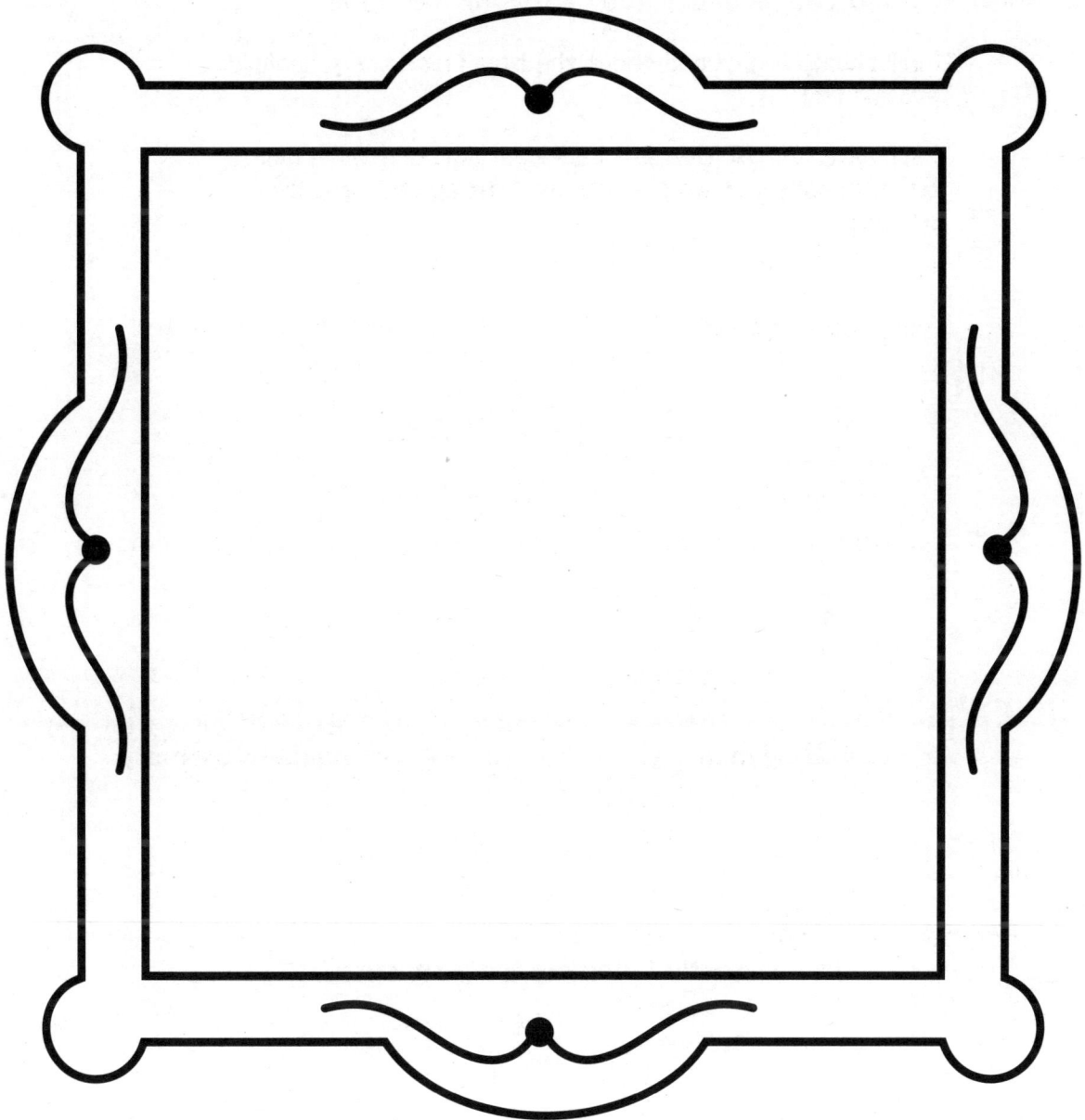

The Memories That Make Me

All of our memories and experiences—even the ones we would rather forget—make us who we are. For this activity, take a moment to think about what life was like, and what you were like, when you were little (exactly how young is up to you). Use the boxes below to fill in some of your most important memories. You can draw them, write them, or attach pictures of them—it is up to you, because they are **your** memories.

"I will always feel proud about the time I won the schoolwide spelling bee."
—GISELA, AGE 15

"I will never forget the time I accidentally burned my mom's birthday cake, but we put lots of frosting on it and ate it anyway."
—HAVEN, AGE 12

A very happy memory:	A very funny memory:
A very proud memory:	A very embarrassing memory:
A very frustrating memory:	A very peaceful memory:

Another memory (your choice!)

Five Times I Was Awesome!

Think back on your experiences and name five times that you were awesome. There are no right or wrong answers here—these can be times when you did a great job in your activities, in your schoolwork, in your relationships with your family and friends, or anything else.

> "I trained all summer, and I made the varsity soccer team as a freshman."
> —ANTONIO, AGE 14

> "I played a holiday piano concert for all the residents at my grandmother's assisted living home."
> —SARA, AGE 12

> "I dressed up as Elton John for Halloween. I made my own costume, and everyone loved it."
> —ANA, AGE 16

1. _____

2. _____

3. _____

4. _____

5. _____

Looking at your list above, do these awesome times have anything in common with each other?

_____

_____

_____

What does it feel like to remember these awesome times?

_____

_____

_____

Feeling the Feels (Even the Hard Ones)

It is helpful to understand the kinds of things that can happen that bring your motivation down and how those situations make you feel on the inside. Below are some unpleasant situations that most kids have experienced. For each one, shade in or highlight the emotions that you think the situation would make you feel. For each one, there is an extra circle where you can write in another emotion.

SITUATION: Being criticized

Afraid	Alone	Angry	Anxious	Ashamed	Confused	Embarrassed	Helpless
Hurt	Impatient	Irritated	Lazy	Resentful	Sad	Stupid	

SITUATION: Doing poorly on a test

Afraid	Alone	Angry	Anxious	Ashamed	Confused	Embarrassed	Helpless
Hurt	Impatient	Irritated	Lazy	Resentful	Sad	Stupid	

SITUATION: Getting blamed or punished for doing something

Afraid	Alone	Angry	Anxious	Ashamed	Confused	Embarrassed	Helpless
Hurt	Impatient	Irritated	Lazy	Resentful	Sad	Stupid	

SITUATION: **Not getting recognized or complimented when you tried hard on something**

Afraid	Alone	Angry	Anxious	Ashamed	Confused	Embarrassed	Helpless
Hurt	Impatient	Irritated	Lazy	Resentful	Sad	Stupid	

SITUATION: **Spending more time than you meant to on video games or social media**

Afraid	Alone	Angry	Anxious	Ashamed	Confused	Embarrassed	Helpless
Hurt	Impatient	Irritated	Lazy	Resentful	Sad	Stupid	

SITUATION: **Bottling your feelings up inside**

Afraid	Alone	Angry	Anxious	Ashamed	Confused	Embarrassed	Helpless
Hurt	Impatient	Irritated	Lazy	Resentful	Sad	Stupid	

SITUATION: **Not knowing how to do something**

Afraid	Alone	Angry	Anxious	Ashamed	Confused	Embarrassed	Helpless
Hurt	Impatient	Irritated	Lazy	Resentful	Sad	Stupid	

Feeling the Feels
(Especially the Good Ones)

It is also helpful—and maybe even more helpful—to know the kinds of situations that bring happiness and how those situations make you feel on the inside. As you did before, shade in or highlight the emotions that you think each situation would make you feel. For each one, there is an extra circle where you can write in another emotion.

SITUATION: **Winning an award**

Accom-plished	Calm	Capable	Centered	Cheerful	Delighted	Energized	Excited
Grateful	Hopeful	Proud	Resilient	Secure	Seen by others	Upbeat	

SITUATION: **Being elected or chosen for a position**

Accom-plished	Calm	Capable	Centered	Cheerful	Delighted	Energized	Excited
Grateful	Hopeful	Proud	Resilient	Secure	Seen by others	Upbeat	

SITUATION: **Getting a good grade on something you worked hard on**

Accom-plished	Calm	Capable	Centered	Cheerful	Delighted	Energized	Excited
Grateful	Hopeful	Proud	Resilient	Secure	Seen by others	Upbeat	

SITUATION: **Getting a compliment**

| Accom-plished | Calm | Capable | Centered | Cheerful | Delighted | Energized | Excited |
| Grateful | Hopeful | Proud | Resilient | Secure | Seen by others | Upbeat | |

SITUATION: **Buying something you wanted with your own money**

| Accom-plished | Calm | Capable | Centered | Cheerful | Delighted | Energized | Excited |
| Grateful | Hopeful | Proud | Resilient | Secure | Seen by others | Upbeat | |

SITUATION: **Spending one-on-one time with your favorite relative**

| Accom-plished | Calm | Capable | Centered | Cheerful | Delighted | Energized | Excited |
| Grateful | Hopeful | Proud | Resilient | Secure | Seen by others | Upbeat | |

SITUATION: **Having extra time to do your favorite activity**

| Accom-plished | Calm | Capable | Centered | Cheerful | Delighted | Energized | Excited |
| Grateful | Hopeful | Proud | Resilient | Secure | Seen by others | Upbeat | |

Seeing Stars

Think about the celebrities, athletes, leaders, or other people you admire or whom you'd like to be like when you are older. Print or copy and paste pictures into the frames below (or, if you feel like flexing different creative muscles, draw pictures or write their names in fancy script).

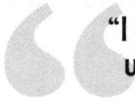

"I really admire all the charity work John Cena has done for kids who are ill."
—PABLO, AGE 12

"I really admire how creative Dolly Parton is. She has written so many songs!"
—HARPER, AGE 15

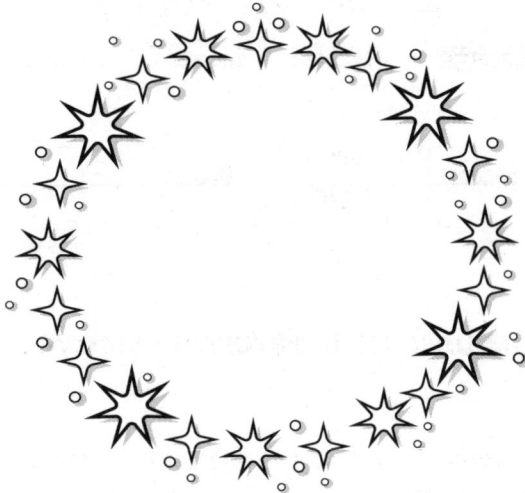

What do you admire most about this person?

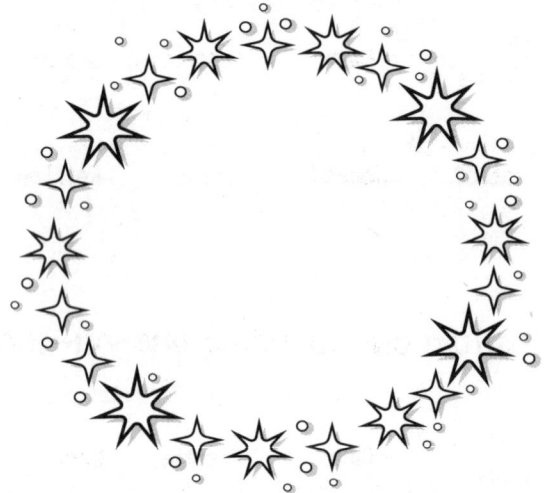

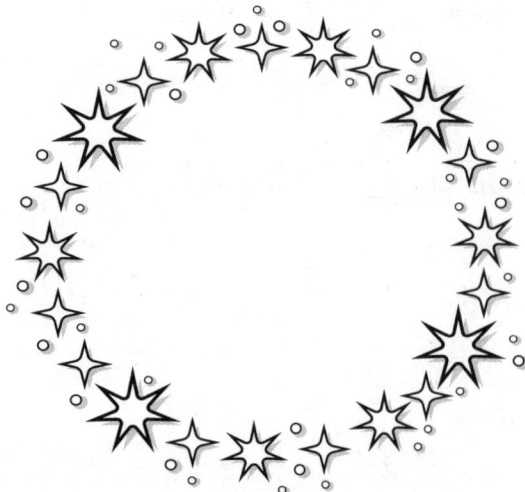

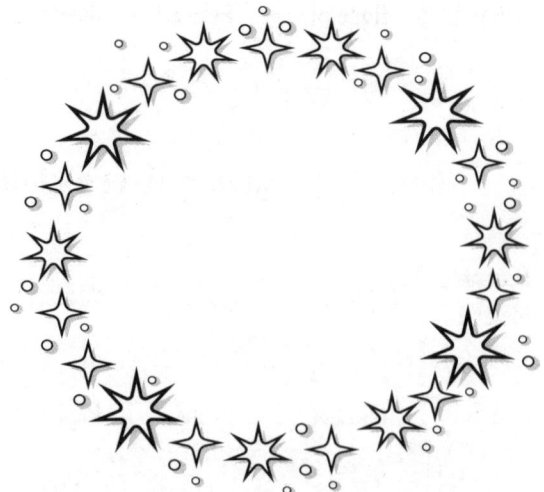

What do you admire most about this person?

What do you admire most about this person?

What do you admire most about this person?

Mottos and Mantras

Do you have a favorite quote or saying that motivates you? If so, write it in fancy letters below. If you are not sure, try searching online for quotes by the stars you identified in "Seeing Stars" (page 28). If you do not find any quotes that "speak" to you, try coming up with your own.

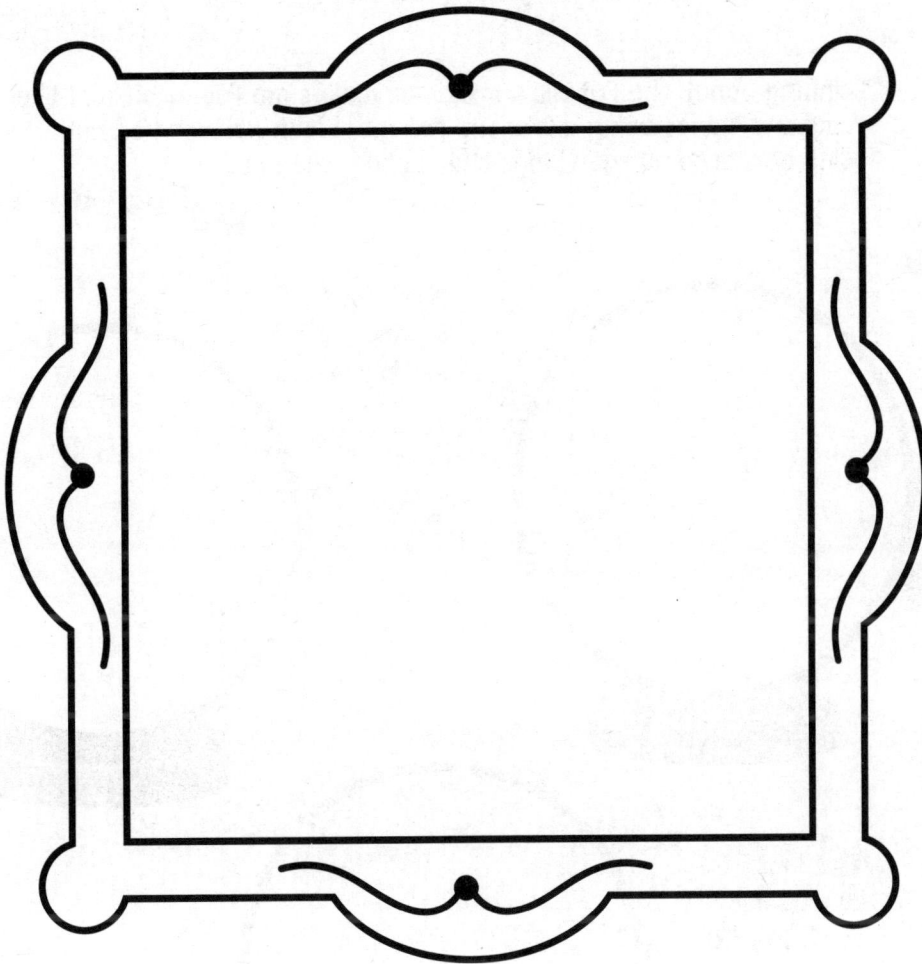

Think about ways you can keep your guiding quote handy and see it often. Could you make it the lock screen on your phone? Could you write it on the cover of your favorite notebook? Or on a sticky note on the bathroom mirror or your instrument case? Try to think about the situations where you most need a boost to keep going.

Peeking into the Future

Imagine your future self! Fill in the crystal balls below with pictures, drawings, or words of the future you.

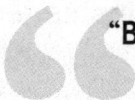

"By next year, I hope I will have published a poem."

—ARIELLA, AGE 14

"In 5 years, I hope I will be playing lacrosse in college."

—MARCO, AGE 16

"Thinking about the future sometimes makes me feel excited. I like imagining things being different for me. I look forward to not being bothered by the things that bother me now."

—KWAMI, AGE 16

What I want
next year
to look like:

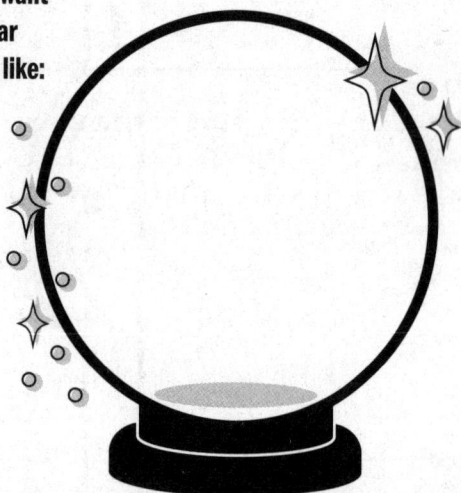

What I want
5 years from
now to look like:

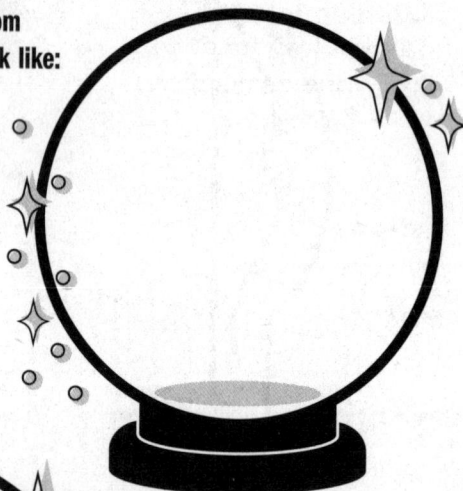

What I want
10 years from
now to look like:

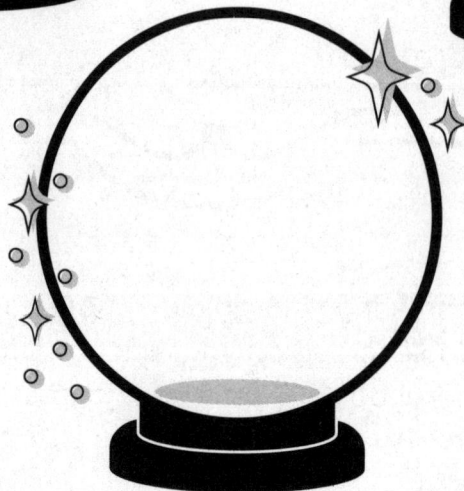

Getting Personal with Personality

One of the main ways we think about personality is with the Big Five personality traits. These are extraversion, neuroticism, openness to experience, conscientiousness, and agreeableness. We know, that's a lot of jargon, and you might not know what all of these things mean—yet. This activity is meant to help you learn more about this way of thinking about personality and to help you figure out where you fall on each trait. On each line below, insert an **X** where you think you would fall on the spectrum from low to high.

> "I like taking quizzes and learning more about my personality. There definitely isn't one right kind of personality to have. Everyone is different." —SARI, AGE 14
>
> "There are lots of different ways to be a person." —EZRA, AGE 15

Extraversion

What low extraversion sounds like:	**What high extraversion sounds like:**
"I like to keep to myself and observe, instead of always putting myself out there. I get my energy from spending time by myself."	"I am friendly and outgoing, and I love spending time with my friends. I can get pretty sad when I do not get to be with my people."

Neuroticism

What low neuroticism sounds like:	**What high neuroticism sounds like:**
"I feel pretty confident in most situations. I know I could handle a lot of things if I had to, so I really do not worry too much."	"I feel stressed and worried about a lot of different things. People tell me not to worry so much, but I cannot seem to turn it off."

Openness to experience

What low openness to experience sounds like:

"I feel comfortable when I do things that are familiar to me. I do not like trying new things, and I definitely do not like taking risks."

What high openness to experience sounds like:

"I love coming up with new ideas and trying new things. It is fun and exciting to take risks and have adventures."

Conscientiousness

What low conscientiousness sounds like:

"I care a lot more about the big picture than all the little details. I do not stress much about my work being perfect."

What high conscientiousness sounds like:

"I care a lot about being organized and careful when I am doing things. I am proud of my work and I hate making mistakes."

Agreeableness

What low agreeableness sounds like:

"I usually think about things in a critical and rational kind of way. I am not afraid of disagreeing with people or doing my own thing."

What high agreeableness sounds like:

"I like getting along with others and keeping the peace. I hate conflict, and I feel really uncomfortable when I disagree with someone."

Field Trip! . . . to the VIA Institute on Character

For this activity, we'd like you to (temporarily!) press pause on your work in this workbook and go online to the VIA Institute on Character.

VIA stands for "Values in Action," and the "values" include 24 different character strengths that are common to people all over the world.

To take the VIA Youth Survey, go to this website: *https://viacharacter.org/account/register*, which will lead you to sign up for an account. (If you are under 13, you will need a parent to do this for you.) Then click on the button that says "Take the Free Survey" to take the survey that is right for your age. Have fun and be honest! When you finish taking the survey, your results will come automatically to your email. Look closely at your top five character strengths. Use that information to answer the questions below:

> "I was kind of surprised to learn that zest is my top character strength. But, now that I think about it, it explains why I like doing and trying a lot of different things—even things that other kids don't understand or seem too afraid to do."
> —ADDISON, AGE 13

#1 character strength: _____

How surprising was this to you?

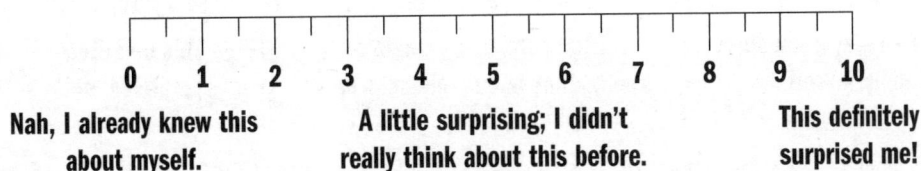

```
  0   1   2   3   4   5   6   7   8   9   10
```

Nah, I already knew this about myself.   **A little surprising; I didn't really think about this before.**   **This definitely surprised me!**

When was there a time that you showed this strength? Write about it or draw/paste in a picture:

#2 character strength: _____

How surprising was this to you?

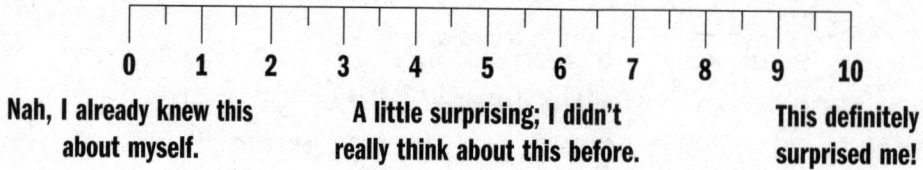

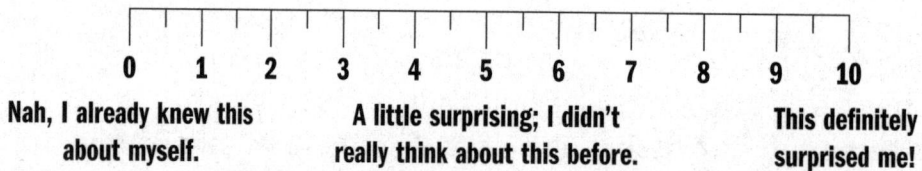

```
0   1   2   3   4   5   6   7   8   9   10
```

Nah, I already knew this   A little surprising; I didn't   This definitely
about myself.   really think about this before.   surprised me!

When was there a time that you showed this strength? Write about it or draw/paste in a picture:

[ ]

#3 character strength: _____

How surprising was this to you?

```
0   1   2   3   4   5   6   7   8   9   10
```

Nah, I already knew this   A little surprising; I didn't   This definitely
about myself.   really think about this before.   surprised me!

When was there a time that you showed this strength? Write about it or draw/paste in a picture:

[ ]

#4 character strength: _____

How surprising was this to you?

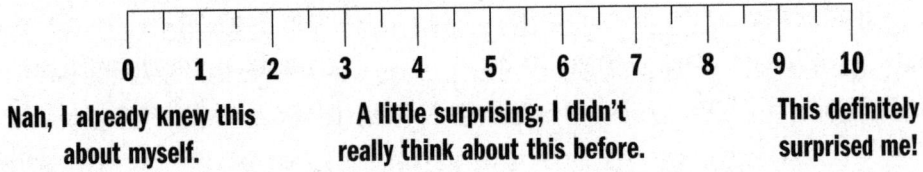

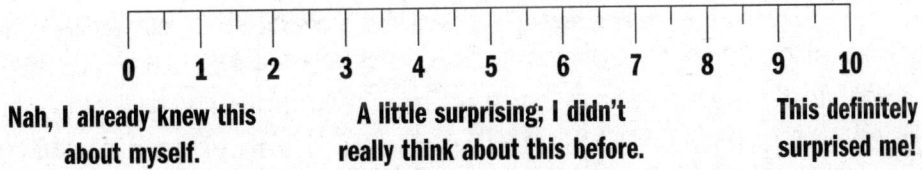

```
0   1   2   3   4   5   6   7   8   9   10
```
**Nah, I already knew this
about myself.**   **A little surprising; I didn't
really think about this before.**   **This definitely
surprised me!**

When was there a time that you showed this strength? Write about it or draw/paste in a picture:

[ ]

#5 character strength: _____

How surprising was this to you?

```
0   1   2   3   4   5   6   7   8   9   10
```
**Nah, I already knew this
about myself.**   **A little surprising; I didn't
really think about this before.**   **This definitely
surprised me!**

When was there a time that you showed this strength? Write about it or draw/paste in a picture:

[ ]

Similar Strengths, Different Strengths

We bet you have heard this expression: "The apple doesn't fall far from the tree." This is understood to mean that kids often have a lot in common with their parents. However, this is hardly true for all kids; even kids who do have a lot in common with their families have times in their lives when they feel very different.

For this activity, look back at the previous activity and find your top five character strengths from the VIA Youth Survey. Write them on the lines below. For each one, mark to what extent this strength makes you similar to or different from the rest of your family.

Character strength: | **How similar or different is this from the rest of my family?**

1.

```
0   1   2   3   4   5   6   7   8   9   10
This makes me        This is kind of like my      My family and I are
very different.          family members.        very similar in this way.
```

2.

```
0   1   2   3   4   5   6   7   8   9   10
This makes me        This is kind of like my      My family and I are
very different.          family members.        very similar in this way.
```

3.

```
0   1   2   3   4   5   6   7   8   9   10
This makes me        This is kind of like my      My family and I are
very different.          family members.        very similar in this way.
```

4.

```
0   1   2   3   4   5   6   7   8   9   10
This makes me        This is kind of like my      My family and I are
very different.          family members.        very similar in this way.
```

5.

```
0   1   2   3   4   5   6   7   8   9   10
This makes me        This is kind of like my      My family and I are
very different.          family members.        very similar in this way.
```

How Do You See Me?

Pretend you're the host of your own YouTube channel. Find three people you know and trust and ask them, "What do you think my strengths are?" Write their responses below:

Interviewee 1: _____

1. _____   2. _____

3. _____

Interviewee 2: _____

1. _____   2. _____

3. _____

Interviewee 3: _____

1. _____   2. _____

3. _____

What did doing this activity feel like? Write about it here:

"A lot of the time, it feels like people tell me what I am doing wrong or what I'm not good at. Interviewing my relatives and finding out what they think my strengths are felt different—and nice for a change."
—MARIO, AGE 13

I Am What I Am . . .
and I'm Not What I'm Not

Below is a list of many different personal qualities. **Shade in or highlight** 10 qualities that you think are strengths for you (fill in the blank one if you like). **Cross out** 10 qualities that you do not think you have.

Active	Adventurous	Affectionate	Agreeable	Bewildered	Big-hearted
Boisterous	Bold	Brainy	Bright	Brilliant	Caring
Cautious	Challenging	Charismatic	Charming	Clear-headed	Clever
Clumsy	Cold	Confident	Confused	Conservative	Courageous
Cowardly	Cunning	Cute	Daring	Dependable	Dynamic
Easily influenced	Easily satisfied	Easygoing	Endearing	Energetic	Engaging
Enlightened	Extraverted	Fidgety	Flexible	Foolish	Friendly
Generous	Gifted	Good-humored	Good-natured	Gutsy	Hopeful

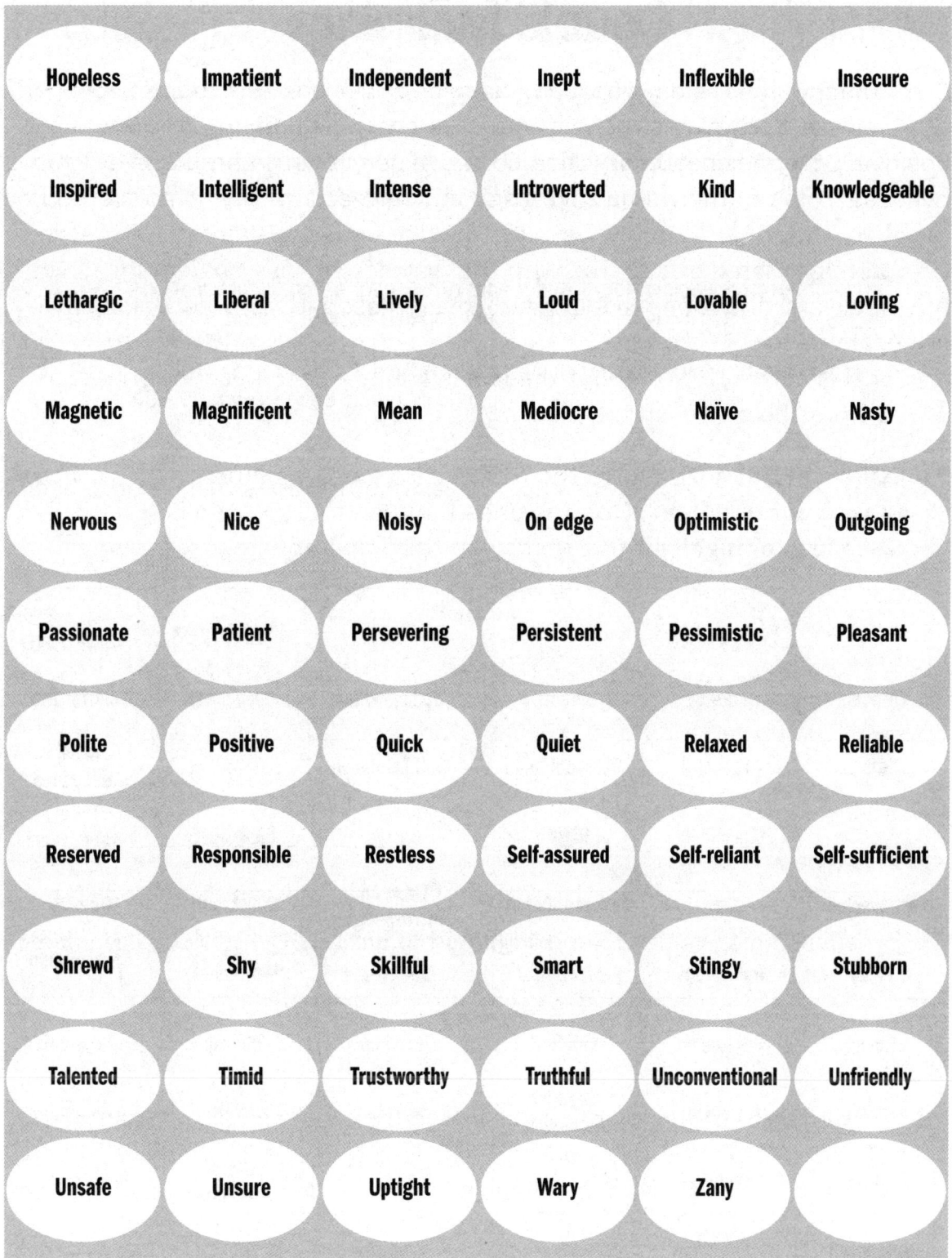

Hopeless	Impatient	Independent	Inept	Inflexible	Insecure
Inspired	Intelligent	Intense	Introverted	Kind	Knowledgeable
Lethargic	Liberal	Lively	Loud	Lovable	Loving
Magnetic	Magnificent	Mean	Mediocre	Naïve	Nasty
Nervous	Nice	Noisy	On edge	Optimistic	Outgoing
Passionate	Patient	Persevering	Persistent	Pessimistic	Pleasant
Polite	Positive	Quick	Quiet	Relaxed	Reliable
Reserved	Responsible	Restless	Self-assured	Self-reliant	Self-sufficient
Shrewd	Shy	Skillful	Smart	Stingy	Stubborn
Talented	Timid	Trustworthy	Truthful	Unconventional	Unfriendly
Unsafe	Unsure	Uptight	Wary	Zany	

Double Meanings

From the day you were born, adults have been using words to describe who you are. Sometimes these labels—like *easygoing, happy,* or *sweet*—are positive. Other descriptions—like *difficult, hyperactive,* and *moody*—are more negative. Lots of other terms, like *quiet* and *relaxed,* are neither positive nor negative. They're just simply ways to describe behavior.

You might agree or disagree with the way adults have characterized you. But labels aren't just one-sided. Nearly every description—whether positive or negative—has an opposite.

For this activity, think about the labels adults use to describe you. Look at the words below (fill in the blank ones if you like) and:

- **Circle or put a ✓** next to the words you've heard before.
- **Cross out or put an X** on the ones that don't fit you at all.
- **Shade in or highlight** the words you think appropriately describe you.

Negative			Positive		
Difficult	Annoying	Hyperactive	Strong-willed	Passionate	Zest for life
Shy	Obsessive	Overanalyzes	Self-reflective	Self-reliant	Social intelligence
Impulsive	Unsociable	Rigid	Curious	Easygoing	Follows rules
Introverted	Slow	Underconfident	Calm and introspective	Consistent	Humble
Picky	Indifferent	Perfectionist	Discerning	Persistent	Appreciation of excellence
Bossy	Outspoken	Inhibited	Determined	Honest	Self-regulated
Tough	Eccentric	Head in the clouds	Resolute	Creative	Hopeful
Distractible	Know-it-all	Class clown	Perceptive	Love of learning	Fun-loving
Unfocused	Overly emotional		Exploring	Values close relationships	

Look at your list. How do you feel about the words you've circled/marked with ✓ or crossed out/marked with **X**?

_____

_____

_____

_____

Are there any words you've both circled/marked with ✓ and highlighted? Write them here:

_____

_____

_____

Are there any words from the negative column that you've highlighted? Write them here:

_____

_____

_____

What would it look like to turn one of your negative labels into its more positive counterpart? Write about it here:

_____

_____

_____

_____

_____

> "People say I am shy, and I think this fits me. I don't think it's necessarily a bad thing, though. Maybe because I am not super outgoing and talking all the time, I notice and think about things that other people miss. I think being quieter on purpose, so that I can pay attention, instead of being quieter out of habit, is the thing that would make me more self-reflective than shy."
> —SABRINA, AGE 16

Fill in the Blank

Below are sentences that have beginnings, but no endings—that part is up to you. For each sentence, make up an ending that is true about you. You can use the list of personal qualities from "I Am What I Am . . . and I'm Not What I'm Not" (pages 38–39) to give you ideas, but it is also fine to come up with your own answers.

I am almost always _____.

I wish I were more _____.

My friends think I am _____.

My parents think I am _____.

My teachers think I am _____.

People who don't know me well think I am _____.

People would be surprised to know that I am _____.

I could never be _____.

When I am older, I want to be _____.

Sometimes I am _____.

My life would be better if only I were _____.

Adults are _____.

My parents are _____.

My friends are _____.

My teachers are _____.

The people I go to school with are _____.

People tell me I should be more _____.

I hope I will always be _____.

Up in My Head

The way we think and talk to ourselves matters a lot. While talking to ourselves in a kind and positive way can be great for boosting motivation, kids sometimes find this awkward or hard to do. Many kids have a "loud inner critic" and are used to talking to themselves in a pretty harsh way.

What kinds of things do you say or think when you are trying to motivate yourself? Some thought bubbles below are already filled in to get you started. If you do not think the thought in the bubble, scribble, strikethrough, or shade it out! Fill in the other bubbles with your own thoughts.

This essay might be annoying, but I know I can do this.

Ugh, I wish I weren't so lazy.

I know I'll feel more at ease once my room is clean.

If I don't practice now, I'm not going to do well, and everyone will judge me.

Once I get started, I know the rest will be pretty easy to do.

What do you notice about the way you talk to yourself? Insert an **X** to mark it on the ruler:

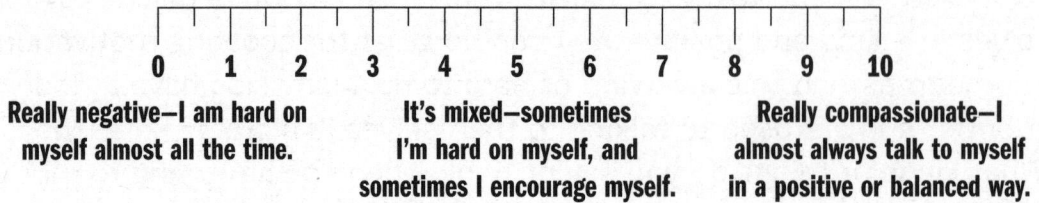

0 1 2 3 4 5 6 7 8 9 10

Really negative—I am hard on myself almost all the time.

It's mixed—sometimes I'm hard on myself, and sometimes I encourage myself.

Really compassionate—I almost always talk to myself in a positive or balanced way.

How well are your thoughts working for you? Insert an **X** to mark it on the ruler:

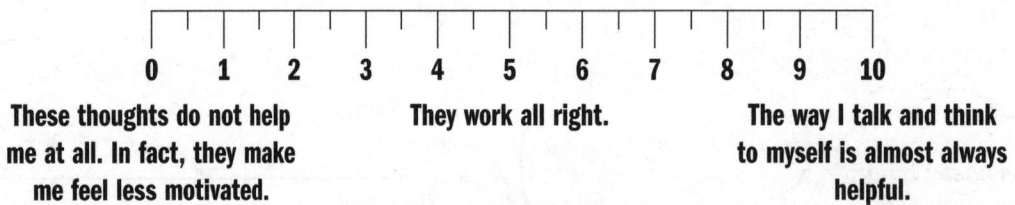

0 1 2 3 4 5 6 7 8 9 10

These thoughts do not help me at all. In fact, they make me feel less motivated.

They work all right.

The way I talk and think to myself is almost always helpful.

Is changing the way you talk to yourself important to you? Insert an **X** to mark it on the ruler:

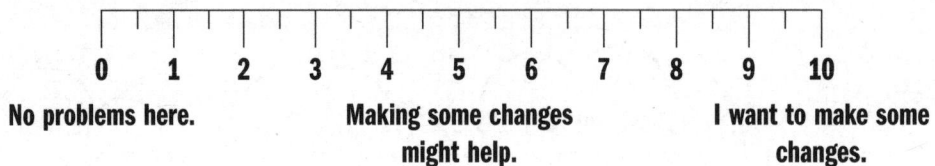

0 1 2 3 4 5 6 7 8 9 10

No problems here.

Making some changes might help.

I want to make some changes.

Too High, Too Low, or Just Right?

Setting the "bar" at the right height is an important part of motivation. Setting expectations too high to reach is a motivation crusher. But when expectations are low, you might not feel like you have a good reason to do anything more than the bare minimum.

Of course, the bars we set for ourselves are important, but the bars that other people set affect us too. The goal of this activity is to identify different areas where the adults in your life set expectations for you. Do their expectations feel too high, too low, or just right?

> "My parents put a lot of pressure on me to play basketball and to get a college scholarship. I like playing, but I'm not as serious about it as they are. I'm also more realistic. They don't understand how playing sports in college works." —LENOX, AGE 15

> "I wish my parents were more supportive of my acting. They never say it directly, but their little comments make it clear that they don't think it's worth my time." —GABRIEL, AGE 13

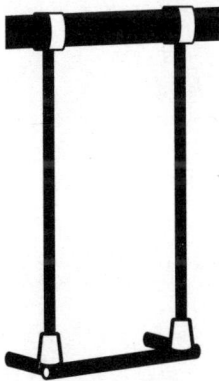

Areas where others' expectations are too high:

_____

_____

_____

How does this feel to you?

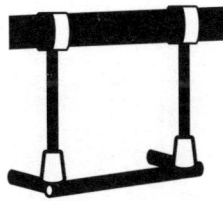

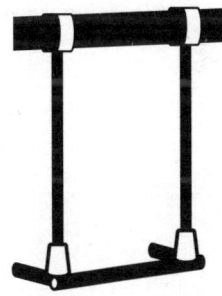

_____

_____

_____

Areas where others' expectations are too low:

_____

_____

_____

How does this feel to you?

_____

_____

_____

Areas where others' expectations are just right:

_____

_____

_____

How does this feel to you?

_____

_____

_____

OK Is OK

It would be amazing if we had unlimited time, energy, and resources to do all the things we do incredibly well. But, for many reasons, not everything can be a top priority (because if everything is a priority, nothing is). This exercise helps you identify activities or areas in your life where you are "just OK" and figure out if this works for you or if you want to change "just OK" into something different.

"I am just OK at playing soccer, but it's really important to my parents that I keep playing on the team. I wish I could stop playing soccer and have that time to do other things I enjoy more."
—OSCAR, AGE 15

An activity or area where you are "just OK":	Is it OK that this is "just OK," or is this something you would like to change?	Do other people in your life (like your parents or teachers) agree or disagree with you about this?

I Wish My Parents Knew . . .

Often there are things that kids wish their parents knew or understood about them. Take a moment and think about the things you wish your parents understood about you. Feel free to write, draw, or paste in pictures, or express yourself in another way.

> "I wish my parents knew how stressful it is when they get overinvolved in my schoolwork."
> —ALAINA, AGE 16

> "I wish my parents knew how much I love them, even though we argue a lot."
> —MIKA, AGE 14

. . . what my life is like when I am with my friends:	. . . what it's like for me when I am doing homework:
. . . what it's like for me when they put pressure on me:	. . . what my life is like when I am at school:
. . . what it's like for me when I feel like I've disappointed them:	. . . something else I wish they could understand about me:

I Wish My Teachers Knew . . .

Often there are things that kids wish their teachers knew or understood about them. Take a moment and think about the things you wish your teacher understood about you. Feel free to write, draw, or paste in pictures, or express yourself in another way. There are some prompts in the boxes below to get you started. The last box invites you to add your own.

"**I wish my teachers knew how much it hurts my feelings when they say I'm not focused.**"
—AVA, AGE 14

. . . what it's like for me when I am in class:

. . . what it's like for me when I am doing homework:

. . . what it's like for me when I am taking a test or quiz:

. . . what it's like for me when I have to give a presentation or talk in class:

. . . what my life is like when I am not at school:

. . . something else I wish they could understand about me:

Where Is My Aptitude Right Now?

In this chapter you completed many activities to help you think about who you are as a person and where your many strengths lie. You also completed activities to help you understand where your strengths do *not* lie, and this is important information too. Based on what you learned about yourself and your aptitudes, fill in the lines below:

Aptitude

Pleasure

Areas where my skills are strong (and may become even stronger):

_____

_____

_____

_____

_____

_____

_____

_____

_____

_____

Practice

3
What Makes Me Happy?

In this chapter you have a chance to take a deep dive into what gives us pleasure. Although you might think this topic was already covered in the worksheets in Chapter 2 that help kids figure out what they're good at, what we're good at doing and what makes us happy aren't always the same. The difference between aptitude and pleasure is that pleasure implies children are doing those activities with enjoyment. Many unmotivated kids either don't know what gives them pleasure or are stuck doing things they're good at doing but that don't make them happy. For example, Maya was great at soccer. She spent 6 years playing soccer on a travel team, but by the time she was 14 years old, she was tired of the sport. Although she was the best player on the team, she didn't enjoy it anymore. Her parents insisted she continue playing, and she reacted by giving up on almost everything. Unfortunately, her life—and the life of her family—had revolved around soccer and she had trouble figuring out how to fill her time with something she enjoyed doing.

It *should* be easy to figure out what makes us happy, but in reality *it's not that easy.* "Do what makes you happy" is a popular piece of advice to college graduates, but what exactly does that mean? We adults aren't that good at identifying the things that make us happy, and often even if we know what makes us happy, we don't spend a lot of time doing those things. No wonder it's hard for kids! Kids have little trouble figuring out what is boring. It's much more difficult for them to engage in discussions about what gives them joy.

This chapter is all about helping kids answer the questions "What gives you pleasure?" and "What makes you happy?" The chapter starts with activities that help kids identify their favorite things, the activities that are fun for them, and the times in their lives when they felt at their best (pages 52–56). Some activities help them identify the things that get in the way of pleasure (page 57) and ways to increase their daily and weekly pleasure (pages 58–64). The last group of activities (pages 65–67) helps them develop a sense of gratitude. Feeling gratitude is an essential skill associated with many positive psychological and health benefits, such as improved sleep, reduced depression, and higher self-esteem. Often the things we are thankful for are also things that bring us pleasure. For kids who have trouble recognizing what gives them pleasure, focusing on gratitude can help them identify specific activities that bring them joy. Developing a regular gratitude practice can also help kids stay engaged when motivation inevitably starts to ebb.

These Are a Few of My Favorite Things

What brings you pleasure? What things make you happy? On the lines below, write down different things that bring you a lot of fun when you get to do them. These can be anything! Then use the ruler to mark and rate how much pleasure it brings you.

Hint: If it feels hard to get started on this activity, try thinking about things that you can notice with your senses (like things that smell good or taste good). You can also look at your work on "Here I Am" (page 21) for ideas.

"**I like looking at pictures from when I was little.**"
—AURORA, AGE 14

_____

0 1 2 3 4 5 6 7 8 9 10

_____

0 1 2 3 4 5 6 7 8 9 10

_____

0 1 2 3 4 5 6 7 8 9 10

_____

0 1 2 3 4 5 6 7 8 9 10

_____

0 1 2 3 4 5 6 7 8 9 10

_____

0 1 2 3 4 5 6 7 8 9 10

Feeling Fun

Sometimes, when our motivation is running low, it can be hard to remember what pleasure feels like. Yet we know that emotions are made up of three main parts—thoughts, behaviors, and body cues—and what *fun* feels like for you is important information for you to have. Use the sketch below to color (or describe with words) and show what it **feels like in your body** when you are having fun. There are no rules here—how you show it is up to you.

Hint: If you have trouble getting started on this one, jump to "When Was the Last Time I Had Fun?" on page 55 and then come back to this one. What does it feel like when you think about having fun?

"When I am having fun, my brain feels warm and sparkly."
—JENNA, AGE 11

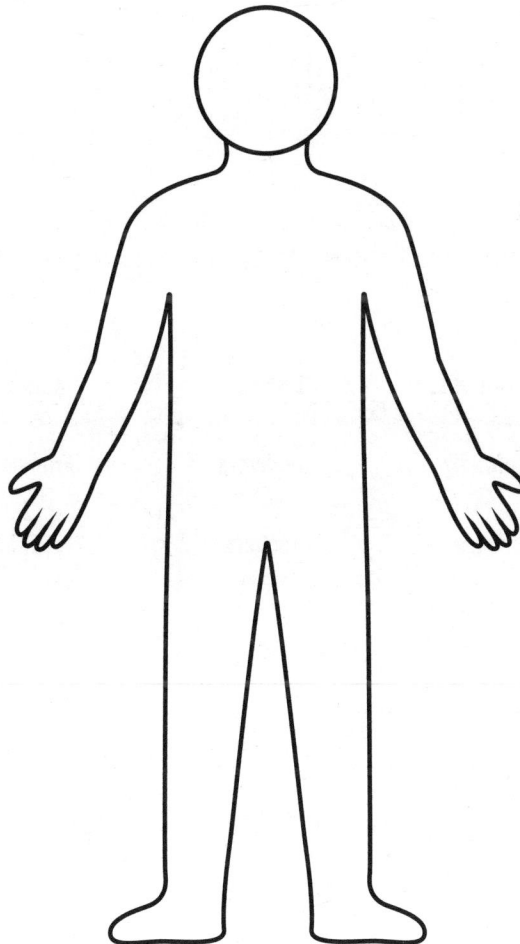

My Favorite Age

The past is full of rich information that you can use to make your *right now* better. For this activity, think about the time in your life when you felt your happiest.

My favorite age was when I was: _____

Include pictures, sketches, cartoons, or words about you that represent what it was like when you were your favorite age:

It was a happy time because of the people I was with, like my . . . (please **shade in or highlight**)

Parents	Grandparents	Siblings	Aunts	Uncles
Cousins	Stepfamily	Neighbors	Friends	Teammates
Boyfriend/girlfriend	Coaches	Teachers	Therapist	Youth group

My favorite things to do were . . .

_____

_____

Nowadays, it makes me feel like my favorite age again when I . . .

_____

_____

When Was the Last Time I Had Fun?

The kinds of activities and situations that were enjoyable for you before can hold a lot of information about what is fun for you now. In this activity, think about the last time you really enjoyed yourself. The questions below help you reflect on why it was as much fun as it was and whether there are ways of experiencing that fun again.

> **"The last time I had a lot of fun was when I won tickets to see my favorite band. I'll never forget that night!"** —AARON, AGE 16
>
> **"The last time I had a lot of fun was when I made jewelry using the new supplies I got for my birthday."** —CAMILA, AGE 13

The last time I had a lot of fun, I was at . . .

_____

_____

And I was with . . .

_____

_____

And I was doing . . .

_____

_____

I think I WILL / WILL NOT (**circle or highlight** one) do this again because . . .

_____

_____

Sometimes people know what they would like to do, but for different reasons it is hard for them to turn that knowledge about it into a plan they can carry out. This is true even for making plans that are fun. If this sounds like you, look ahead to the activity "Turning Ideas into Action Plans" (pages 112–113).

Surprising Fun!

We are often very good at predicting the things we will enjoy and the things we will not. Sometimes, though, fun can take us by surprise. This can give us new information about who we are and what we like (and what we don't like, which is important information too). For each of the prompts below, write a few words or draw or paste in a picture (or an emoji!) to remind yourself about each time this has happened to you.

> "I was really excited to go snowboarding for the first time, but I spent the whole day falling down on my butt! It ended up being hard, painful, and not much fun for me, even though I know lots of kids really like it, and I thought I would too. I'm probably not going to go snowboarding again, but I'm glad I tried it."
> —SIMON, AGE 16

A time that you thought something was going to be very fun . . . and it turned out to be just as fun as you'd thought:

A time that you thought something was not going to be very fun . . . but it turned out to be more fun than you'd expected:

A time that you thought something was going to be very fun . . . but it turned out not to be as much fun as you'd thought:

A time that you thought something was not going to be fun . . . and you were totally right—it wasn't fun at all:

Don't Marsh My Mellow!

Unfortunately, a lot of things can get in the way of having fun or make fun times less fun. Can you identify some of the things that marsh your mellow? Write them in below.

> "It always bugs me when my dad asks me about doing my homework as soon as I'm home from school. I need to relax first!"
> —JAMES, AGE 15

> "Sometimes when I am with my friends, I start thinking about all the work I need to do for school, and that doesn't feel so good."
> —ALEX, AGE 13

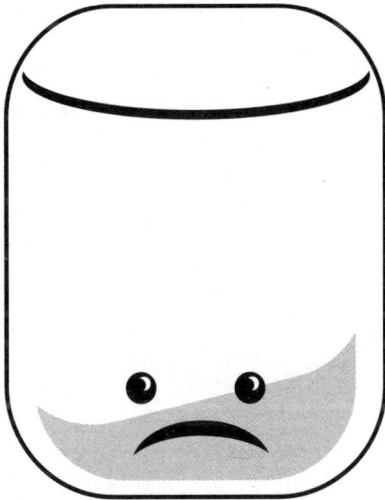
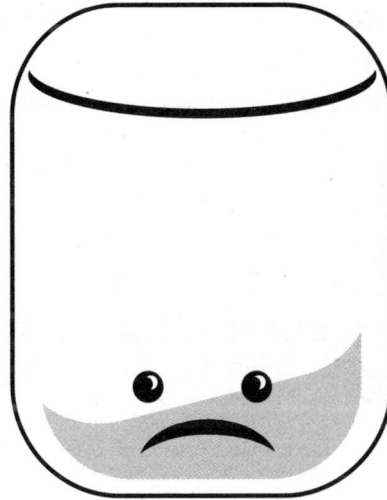
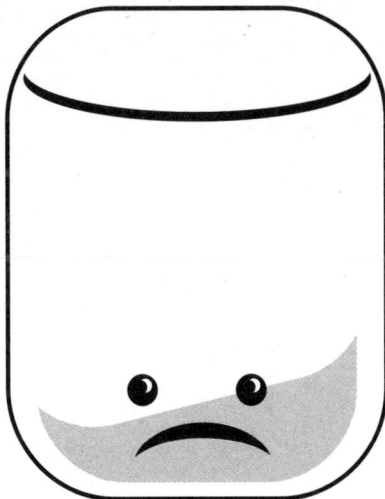
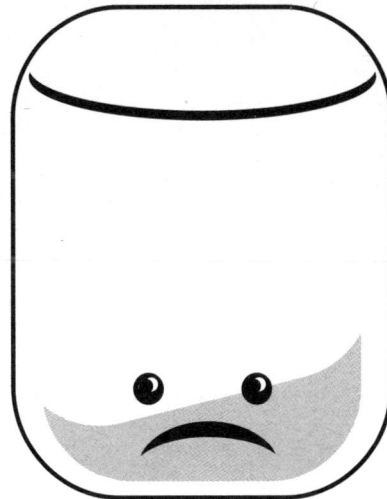

Best. Day. Ever.

Imagine what it would feel like to have the best day EVER. Try not to focus too much on what's possible and what isn't—for this activity, the sky's the limit!

> "On my best day ever, I would go with my two best friends to this cool place near my apartment where they have indoor mini-golf and Ping Pong. I'd eat lots of pizza and ice cream, and I wouldn't think about any stressful stuff at all." —LOGAN, AGE 13

Where I would go:	What I would do during the day:	What I would do during the evening:
Who I would spend time with:	What I would eat and drink:	What I would think about:

Use the space below to picture your best day ever. You can write about it, draw it, or paste in pictures to make a collage.

Put an **X** on the rule to mark how often you currently get to do the things that would be part of your best day ever:

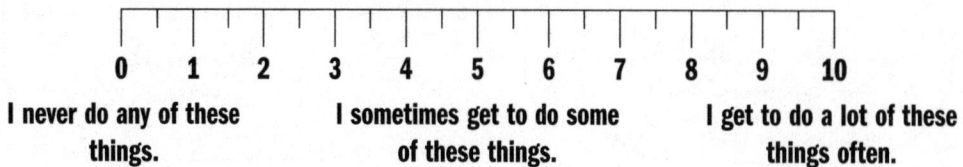

```
    0   1   2   3   4   5   6   7   8   9   10
```

I never do any of these things.   I sometimes get to do some of these things.   I get to do a lot of these things often.

Best Day Ever—With a Twist

Look back at the fun ideas you came up with in "Best. Day. Ever." (page 58). This activity is meant to challenge you to think of some new ideas for having fun. Often, working within constraints or boundaries (like the ones the questions below give you) helps people tap into their creativity and discover new ideas and solutions.

What would a really fun day look like if . . . you weren't able to use any screens or technology for the whole day?

"I would pack a picnic with all my favorite foods, and I would go fishing and day camping in the woods."
—HANNAH, AGE 14

What would a really fun day look like if . . . you could only spend $10?

"I would go to the library in my town, find a comfy chair, and read a bunch of graphic novels."
—FELIX, AGE 12

What would a really fun day look like if . . . you couldn't travel farther than one block from where you live?

"I would invite my friends over to my house for a glow-in-the-dark dance party."
—IRIS, AGE 15

What would a really fun day look like if . . . you couldn't spend any of the day at home?

"I would ask my aunt to take me on a road trip to a town I've never been to before."
—THEO, AGE 14

What would a really fun day look like if . . . you had to spend the whole day by yourself?

"I would rewatch the TV shows that I used to like when I was little."
—NOLAN, AGE 16

What would a really fun day look like if . . . you didn't have to follow any of the household rules that you usually have to follow?

"I would probably do the things I was supposed to do anyway, just on my own time frame."
—LIBBY, AGE 14

Keeping a Happiness Calendar

When it comes to creating happiness, having frequent experiences that spark pleasure is often more helpful than having infrequent experiences that bring a LOT of pleasure. This activity helps you find ways to boost your happiness in a simple, day-to-day way. Below are examples of simple pleasures that often make people feel good. Planning for happiness by putting activities like these on your calendar is one way to infuse more fun and happiness into your life.

Examples of mood-boosting activities:

Going to the Dollar Store	Eating a piece of candy	Giving your pet extra attention
Having a phone or video call with your favorite relative	Doing a craft project	Cooking or baking something
Painting, coloring, or drawing	Walking to a convenience store to get a treat	Rereading a favorite book
Painting your fingernails or toenails (or getting someone else to do it for you!)	Styling your hair in a different way from usual	Watching an online tutorial to do fancy makeup
Going to an arcade to play different video games	Looking at old pictures or videos from when you were little	Looking at old artwork or schoolwork that you did when you were little
Playing catch with a friend or family member	Making slime	Making a greeting card for someone else
Planning for a special event	Going to a library or used bookstore	Going to a consignment or thrift store
Going to a favorite restaurant for a meal or dessert	Going to a new restaurant that you have been wanting to try	Going to a sporting goods store and looking at and trying out all the equipment
Reading a new magazine	Taking a bath with a bath bomb	Buying and using a new body lotion or scent

What are some of your mood-boosting activities that aren't listed on page 61? If you need help getting started, try looking at your work on "These Are a Few of My Favorite Things" at the beginning of this chapter (page 52).

Making a plan to have fun, putting it on your calendar, and telling other people about your plans are ways to increase the chances of your doing the things that will bring you pleasure. Not having a clear plan can make it a lot easier to forget to do fun stuff or to allow other not-so-fun stuff to crowd out the time you were going to spend having fun. See below for an example of what planning for fun might look like on someone's calendar:

Sun.	Mon.	Tues.	Wed.	Thurs.	Fri.	Sat.
In a.m.: take Trixie for an extra-long walk to the dog park	After school: go to Dollar Store and get new nail polish, bath bombs, and art supplies	In p.m.: mani/pedi with new polish after homework is done	After school: call Aunt Susan	In p.m.: make a card for Gramps's birthday	In p.m.: take a bath with a bath bomb	In afternoon: go to arcade with my friends

What fun events can you put on your calendar? Try filling in the calendar below for yourself:

Sun.	Mon.	Tues.	Wed.	Thurs.	Fri.	Sat.

Same Old, Same Old . . . But Fun This Time

There are a lot of things that kids have to do that definitely aren't that fun, and we bet you can think of a few. There are also lots of things that kids have to do that are pretty neutral—they're not terrible, but they're not really that fun either. Below is a list of ordinary things kids often have to do, as well as a list of ways to make an activity more fun (or at least different from usual). **Your job is to connect one activity from the left column and one option for making it fun from the right column (drawing a line between them or highlighting them) and see what happens.**

Same old, same old . . .	. . . But fun this time
Taking care of a pet (like going for a walk, cleaning a litter box, or giving your pet a bath)	Pretend that you are a sports commentator and give a running commentary (either silently or out loud) on whatever you are doing.
Traveling to and from your school	Pay attention to each one of your senses (sight, smell, taste, touch, and hearing) while you're doing what you're doing, and see what you notice.
Brushing your teeth	Either in your head or out loud, make up a rhyming poem (à la Dr. Seuss) that describes what you are doing.
Taking a bath or shower	Do whatever you're doing in the reverse order of how you'd usually do it.
Picking out your clothes	For 1 minute, try to do the thing you are doing with your eyes closed (so long as it's safe!) and see what happens.
Doing laundry	Try doing the activity with your nondominant hand (using your left hand if you are a righty and vice versa).
Washing the dishes, loading the dishwasher, or putting clean dishes away	Sing a song or play music while doing the activity.

Lighting a Lamp

Doing something helpful or kind for someone (or something) else is an unexpected source of pleasure for many people. Below are some ideas to try out the next time you are having a hard day, need a pleasure boost, are feeling bored, or just because! Use the thermometer to rate how much fun you think each activity would be for you.

Activity	Rating
Take care of a family pet (like taking your dog on an extra walk, giving your dog a bath, or cleaning your cat's litter box).	0 1 2 3 4 5 6 7 8 9 10
Do something to care for your family's living space (like wiping down the counters, unloading the dishwasher, or organizing a cluttered space).	0 1 2 3 4 5 6 7 8 9 10
Text or call a relative just to say "hi."	0 1 2 3 4 5 6 7 8 9 10
Sort through the clothes or toys you don't use anymore and pack them up for donating.	0 1 2 3 4 5 6 7 8 9 10
Write a note to a former teacher, coach, or other adult who means a lot to you.	0 1 2 3 4 5 6 7 8 9 10
Spend extra time with a sibling or younger family member.	0 1 2 3 4 5 6 7 8 9 10
Volunteer at a local organization that accepts and needs drop-in volunteers (like sorting donations and supplies at a food pantry).	0 1 2 3 4 5 6 7 8 9 10
Show a relative or another adult how to use their technology.	0 1 2 3 4 5 6 7 8 9 10
Make something creative (like a picture, photograph, or poem) for someone else.	0 1 2 3 4 5 6 7 8 9 10
Offer to help a neighbor with a household task or chore.	0 1 2 3 4 5 6 7 8 9 10
Do something to benefit your favorite setting (for example, picking up trash at a local park).	0 1 2 3 4 5 6 7 8 9 10

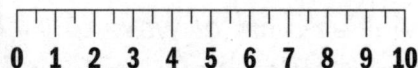

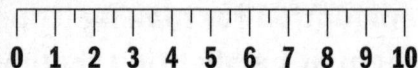

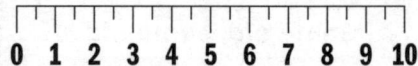

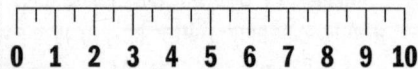

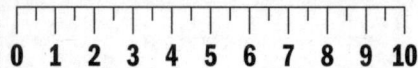

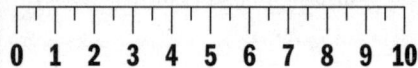

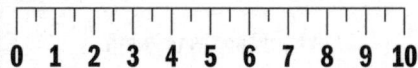

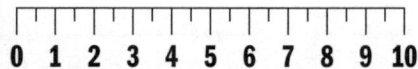

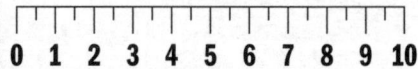

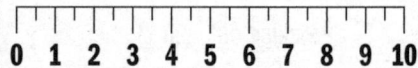

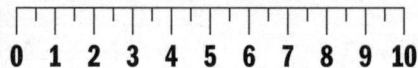

If you feel ready to try one of these activities, go for it! See what you notice when you act in service of someone or something else. If this sounds appealing to you but you're not quite sure how to put it into motion, look ahead to "Turning Ideas into Action Plans" on pages 112–113.

What Is Gratitude?

Research shows us that there are many benefits of incorporating gratitude into daily life. Some people confuse practicing gratitude with toxic positivity ("good vibes only!"). Practicing gratitude is very different. It involves shifting your attention, on purpose, to the things you have, instead of focusing on the things you do not have. Practicing gratitude also has to do with recognizing that things can be beautiful, even when they are hard, and appreciating that bad things, but also great things, happen every day.

Take a moment and think about something you are grateful for. Illustrate or write about it here:

Practicing Gratitude

> "When I went to my grandfather's house for dinner, he made everyone say one thing they were grateful for before the food was served. I acted like I thought it was dumb, but it actually made me less worried about stuff that didn't matter. Nowadays, I try to take a picture every day of something that I'm grateful for. When I'm feeling down or discouraged, I look through my phone, and it helps me focus on what I really want."
>
> —TAREEK, AGE 16

Below are some ways that kids make gratitude a part of their everyday lives. Take a look and color in or highlight the ones that you could see yourself trying, even once:

Taking a picture of something colorful or beautiful

Writing a thank you note or email to someone who has helped you

In a lined notebook, writing down one thing per day that you are grateful for

Keeping a gratitude sketchbook or scrapbook, where you can draw and craft the things you are grateful for

Pausing and taking a quiet moment to visualize something you are grateful for

Before going to bed, thinking about one thing that happened that day that you are grateful for

Finally, we encourage you to plan to practice gratitude at least once a day for a full week. You might choose to practice the same way each day, or this could be an opportunity to experiment with different ways of practicing gratitude to help you figure out what feels right to you. Fill in the worksheet below with your gratitude practice:

Day and date	Time of day	How I practiced gratitude
Monday, February 26	7:00 a.m.	I thought about the things in my life that I'm grateful for while brushing my teeth and washing my face.

After practicing gratitude each day for a full week, what do you notice?

Where Is My Pleasure Right Now?

In this chapter you completed many activities to help you think about where your pleasure comes from and the types of situations and activities where you feel your happiest. Based on what you've learned about yourself and how you feel pleasure, fill in the lines below:

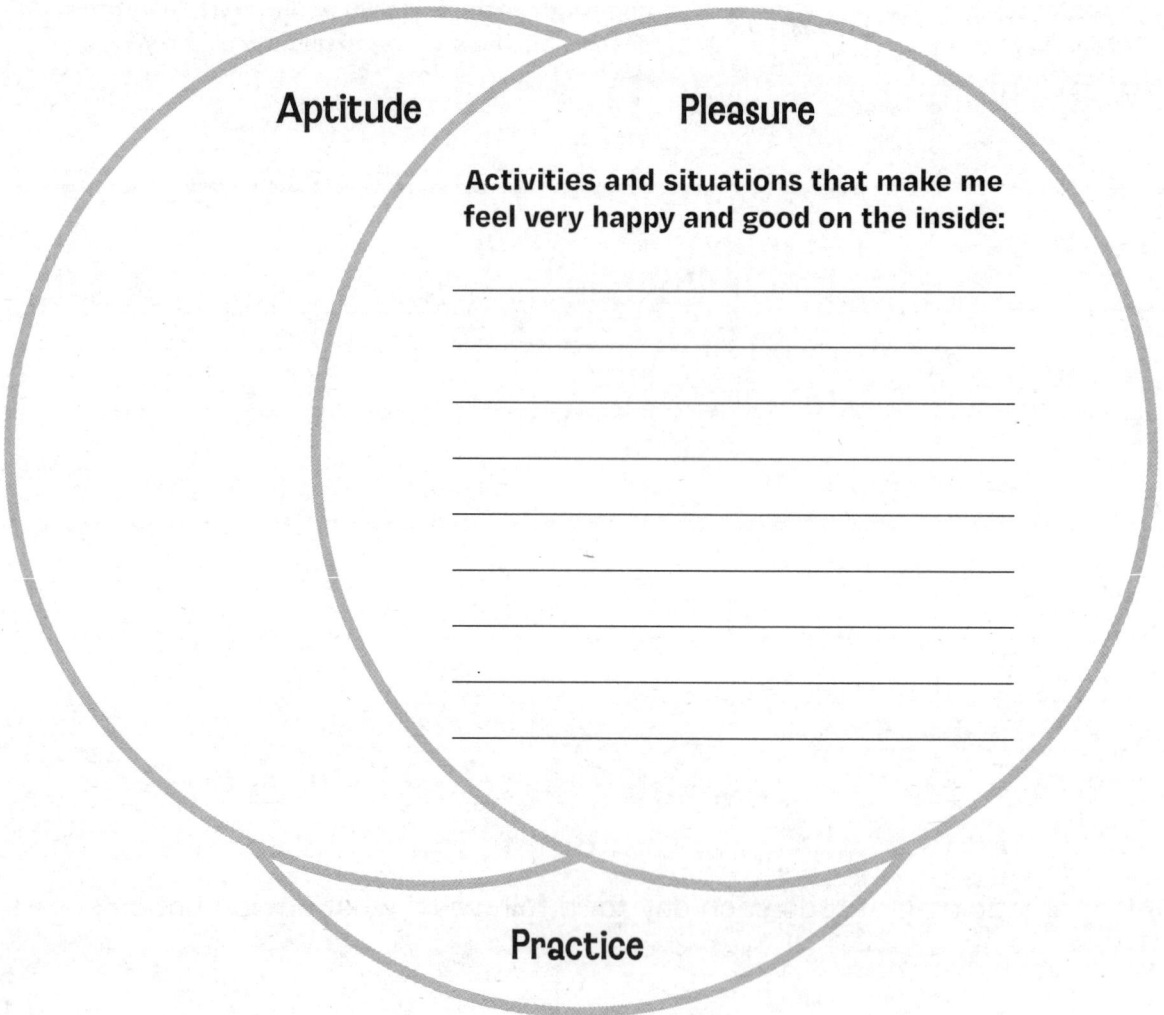

Aptitude

Pleasure

Activities and situations that make me feel very happy and good on the inside:

_____

_____

_____

_____

_____

_____

_____

_____

Practice

4

How Can I Get More of What Makes Me Happy?

This chapter helps kids find ways to spend more time doing what they love. This is the area where aptitude and pleasure combine as a desire to do something. We refer to this skill as *practicing*. *Practice* might bring up negative connotations of multiplication flash cards or clarinet lessons for the sixth-grade orchestra, but what we're referring to here is an activity repeated regularly with intention, sometimes referred to as *deliberate practice*. Deliberate practice is the opposite of rote repetition. It's an intentional, purposeful approach to learning something new or getting better at a skill you've already learned.

Deliberate practice focuses on the *things that are hard.* It's not about doing 10 minutes of math flash cards but about perfecting your free throw if you love to play basketball. For kids, it *requires feedback* from adults in the environment. It *requires concentration,* which means that social media and the phone can't be nearby. It can be helpful to talk to kids about this as being "their time" or what adults might call "me time." Finally, practice isn't a *one-time thing.* Deliberate practice requires, well, practice until you reach mastery. It is goal focused and meaningful.

The activities in this chapter help kids figure out how to spend more time doing meaningful activities. The activities start by asking kids to take note of how they're spending their time. Some activities challenge kids to think about what gets in the way of spending time doing things they love—things such as overscheduling and failures. There are activities that help kids learn to silence their inner critic, to think about when it's OK to give up, how to keep their activities to a reasonable level, and how to handle setbacks. The chapter ends with asking kids to fill out a complete Venn diagram (the diagram introduced at the end of Chapter 1) to help them organize what they've learned about themselves in Chapters 2, 3, and 4 by focusing on the intersection of their aptitudes, pleasures, and what they are interested in spending time practicing.

Spending Time in My Aptitude Zone

It's probably not surprising that most people feel motivated when they get to spend a lot of their time doing things they are good at and enjoy doing. However, for many reasons, kids often feel they must spend a lot of time doing things they do not excel at and do not enjoy either. As you might expect, this is a huge motivation zapper.

You do many different things every day. It's likely that some of these are things you must do and that if you didn't do them there would be negative consequences. However, there is time each day when you have more flexibility. The goal of this activity is to help you think about how you spend your time each day and how these activities line up—or don't line up—with your aptitudes.

Think about a typical **weekday** and write down the activities that you spend the most time doing. Write how long you spend doing each one every day and whether your aptitude for it is high, medium, or low:

Activity	Amount of time spent per day	Your aptitude level (circle or highlight one)
Example: Math (including attending class and completing homework)	2 hours	High (Medium) Low
		High Medium Low
		High Medium Low
		High Medium Low
		High Medium Low
		High Medium Low

Now think about a typical **weekend** or **school holiday** and complete the same worksheet:

Activity	Amount of time spent per day	Your aptitude level (circle or highlight one)
Example: *Shooting baskets at the local basketball court*	*1 hour*	(High) Medium Low
		High Medium Low
		High Medium Low
		High Medium Low
		High Medium Low
		High Medium Low

What do you notice about your responses above? Do you spend more time, less time, or about the right amount of time doing activities that line up with your aptitudes? Think about any changes you can make to spend more time in your "aptitude zone" and write them here:

_____

_____

_____

"Getting a peer math tutor at school was really helpful—it boosted my math skills, which also meant that I was able to do my homework faster."
—GERRY, AGE 14

"I've started waking up half an hour earlier than usual on weekends so that I have some quiet time to work on my paintings, which I really enjoy."
—EMIL, AGE 16

Feeling Overscheduled

Have you ever felt like your schedule was way too packed? Having too many things to do—even if they are things you like doing—is a common motivation zapper for kids and teens. Feeling like you have too little control over your schedule is too. Below are some signs and signals that you might be overscheduled; for each one, place an **X** on the scale to show how often you feel this way:

	This never happens to me.	This sometimes happens to me.	This very often happens to me.
Feeling run down or exhausted		0 1 2 3 4 5 6 7 8 9 10	
Feeling easily annoyed or irritable		0 1 2 3 4 5 6 7 8 9 10	
Feeling happy and excited when things get canceled and you get unexpected free time		0 1 2 3 4 5 6 7 8 9 10	
Having to stay up very late to complete school assignments		0 1 2 3 4 5 6 7 8 9 10	
Feeling like everything is a chore or just something that needs to be checked off your to-do list		0 1 2 3 4 5 6 7 8 9 10	
Being weighed down by thoughts about all the things you have to do		0 1 2 3 4 5 6 7 8 9 10	
Turning in assignments late (or not turning them in at all) because you did not have enough time to do them		0 1 2 3 4 5 6 7 8 9 10	
Having to pull an all-nighter to be ready for the next day's activities		0 1 2 3 4 5 6 7 8 9 10	
Making up excuses to skip activities (especially ones you usually like)		0 1 2 3 4 5 6 7 8 9 10	
Staying up later than you intended to, just to have downtime after you've finished the day's tasks		0 1 2 3 4 5 6 7 8 9 10	

What do you notice about your responses above? Do you think you might be **overscheduled?** If a lot of these signs and signals ring true for you, write one change you could make:

"The next time I'm feeling under the weather, I am going to take a 'personal day' to rest, instead of powering through the way I usually try to do."
—ANASTASIA, AGE 14

Love It, Hate It, or Need a Little Push?

Well-meaning adults often give kids "pushes" or reminders to do many things. While these are sometimes helpful and appreciated, they usually are not. The goal of this activity is to help you take stock of your activities, and to help you—and the adults in your life—figure out how to do "pushes" better.

I've got this!
Activities I can do independently without help from adults

I've kinda got this!
Activities where adults can be helpful, especially when getting started

I don't have this!
Activities that are a lot harder for me to start and finish, where adults often remind me to do this and sometimes their reminders make me feel stressed

Look back at your work on "I Wish My Parents Knew . . . " (page 47) and "I Wish My Teachers Knew . . . " (page 48) for ideas to answer these questions:

For me, a helpful push looks like this: | **And an unhelpful push looks like this:**

"It's not helpful when my dad asks me a million times if I've finished a project or paper. It actually makes it even harder for me to do the work—not easier. It would be nice if we could make plans for after I've finished big projects, and then my dad could remind me about those plans."
—LOUISA, AGE 16

Work It!

Working toward rewards makes it easier for many people to **do the thing.** For example, studying for your driving learner's permit exam might sound boring and tedious, but the reward for studying and passing your exam is that you get to start driving on the road. Sometimes the reward flows naturally from the hard work—like passing your learner's permit exam—but sometimes the reward isn't so straightforward. Sometimes the reward is so far into the future that you might not feel very motivated to do the work now. This activity is meant to help you identify the kinds of rewards that motivate you to do hard things.

Is there a time that you ever earned what felt like a great reward? This could have looked like:

- Being chosen as a captain of a sports team
- Going on a shopping trip after getting high grades on your report card
- Getting a lot of compliments and praise for your performance in the school play
- Having your curfew extended after doing extra chores at home
- . . . or something completely different!

Think about this special reward and illustrate or write about it here:

On the next page are some examples of rewards that kids and teens often find motivating. Circle or highlight the ones that you think would help you work hard.

Getting a "free pass" on chores you'd normally have to do	Earning cash that you can spend however you like	Getting a manicure at a salon	Getting your curfew extended
Getting lots of praise from your teachers	Getting a gift card to your favorite coffee shop	Getting lots of praise from your parents	Getting lots of praise from your friends or classmates
Earning honors or awards from your school	Upgrading your phone or tablet	Earning an academic scholarship	Getting extra screen time or video game time
Getting tickets to see your favorite band in concert	Getting a gift card to your favorite clothing store	Going to an amusement park	Getting to host a special party or event for your friends
Getting to sleep in on a day when you'd normally have to wake up early	Getting your own pet	Going to the movies or having a special movie night at home	Getting new clothes, shoes, or accessories

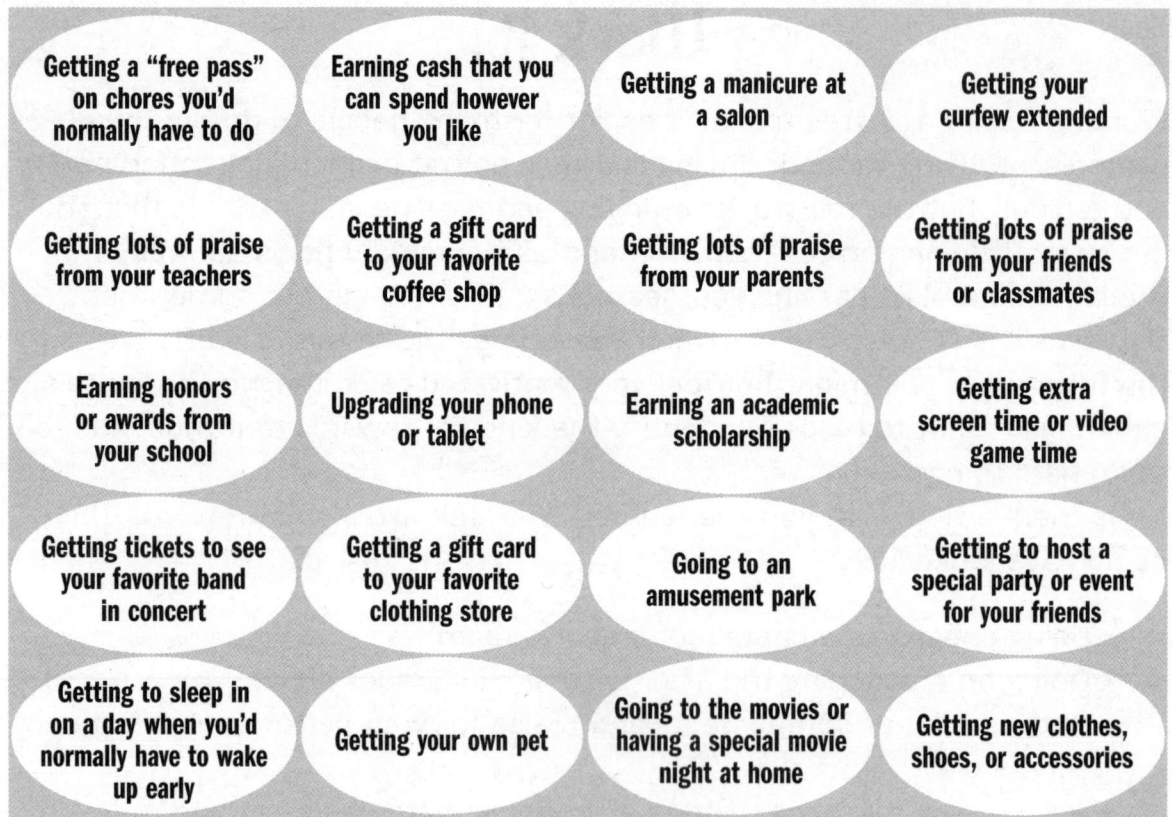

Next, look at the rewards you circled or highlighted and see if you can find any patterns. For example, does the possibility of earning money or items excite you? Or are you motivated to earn chances to do fun things? Or do you find getting a break from some of the things you'd usually be expected to do the most rewarding? Write what you notice here:

_____

_____

Now that you have more information about the kinds of rewards that motivate you, how can you use this to your advantage? Is there anything you have learned about your "reward style" that would be helpful to share with your parents or other people in your life? If this is something you'd like to do but aren't sure where to begin, skip ahead to "Adult Education" on page 111.

_____

_____

_____

Bringing Back the Good

Sometimes it can be difficult to come up with ideas for fun when we're feeling down or especially unmotivated. Fortunately, the activities we enjoyed when we were younger can give us helpful information to use when planning for more fun now. For this activity we would like you to flip back to the activity "My Favorite Age" on page 54.

What were the favorite activities that you came up with?

Are these activities still part of your life? Mark your answer with a ✓ or an **X**.

☐ Yes—definitely!   ☐ No—I've outgrown this stuff.   ☐ Sort of . . .

If you answered "no" or "sort of," is there any way to bring these activities back into your life and enjoy them again? What might this look like?

> "When I was little, I used to love coloring in coloring books with scented markers. Even though I hadn't colored in a really long time, I recently decided to get some scented flair pens and an adult coloring book. I was amazed by how many fun ones there are out there."
> —CRISTINA, AGE 16

> "I used to love making forts with pillows and blankets and hiding out when I was little. Just for fun, I recently made another one and hung out in it all afternoon while I read a book with a flashlight."
> —JORDAN, AGE 14

When a Fail Is a Win

When you don't reach a goal, you might feel disappointed, dejected, angry, or embarrassed. However, as these feelings change, and as more time grows between you and your setback, you might realize things about the situation that you did not notice before. The goal of this activity is to look back on a time that you "failed" and see if there were any helpful things you learned from having it not turn out the way you had planned.

> "I felt really upset and embarrassed when I did not make the dance team at my school. It ended up working out because the dance team members have to go to a lot of trainings and camps during the summer. I ended up getting a summer job that I loved, which I couldn't have done if I'd made the dance team."
> —FARRAH, AGE 16

One of my biggest failures was when . . .

What I was aiming for was . . .

But this is what actually happened . . .

What I learned from going through this is . . .

If I could do it again, I would . . .

When a Win Is a Fail

"Be careful what you're wishing for . . . you might end up getting something you don't want." —UNKNOWN

"I am a decent trombone player, and my parents and music teacher pushed me really hard to try out for All-State Band. I didn't think I would get in, but I did. My parents and music teacher were really excited about it, but they didn't have to go to all the weekend rehearsals like I did. I ended up having a lot less time to myself, and it turned playing music into a stressful thing, which it hadn't been before." —MARTIN, AGE 15

The flip side of having good things grow out of our failures is that sometimes achieving something that we wanted doesn't turn out to be the win we thought it would be. Similarly, sometimes the people in our lives (we're looking at you, adults) might be so impressed or excited by something we did that they end up pushing us to pursue something we were never too excited about in the first place. This activity helps you think about a time when something went well for you but there were hidden consequences.

The people in my life got really excited about the time that I . . .

This is how I felt about my win . . .

I didn't expect the win to have some drawbacks, like . . .

What I learned from going through this is . . .

If I could do it again, I would . . .

Give Me a Break—From Myself!

If you have a loud and judgmental inner critic, this activity is for you. Take a moment to look at some of the critical or negative thoughts you came up with in "Up in My Head" (pages 43–44). What would it be like to turn some of these negative thoughts into more neutral or balanced ones? The first one gives you an example of what this might sound like. Fill in the others with your thoughts from the previous activity, "When a Win Is a Fail."

If I don't practice now, I'm not going to do well and everyone will judge me.

→

Doing my best in the concert matters to me, so I am going to set a timer to start practicing now.

What do you think might happen if you tried out some of these more neutral or balanced thoughts?

How likely do you think you are to try out some of these new thoughts?

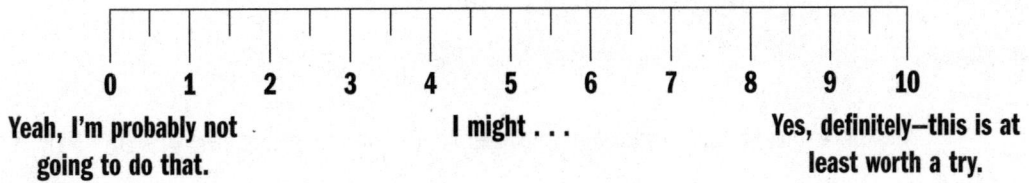

```
  0    1    2    3    4    5    6    7    8    9    10
Yeah, I'm probably not        I might . . .        Yes, definitely—this is at
  going to do that.                                  least worth a try.
```

Break It Down Now

We have all been there: when a task seems way too hard or complicated, it's way too easy to ignore and to avoid getting started. This leads to having even less time to do the hard thing, and stressing about that can make it even harder to get started—you get the picture. Fortunately, one of the best tools we have for breaking this pattern is breaking down big projects into the smallest pieces possible so that they aren't as intimidating anymore. We are willing to bet you have heard this before. But do you know what "breaking it down" actually looks like? Often, breaking it down is a step that needs to be repeated—you might need to keep breaking it down, and breaking it down again, until you have a clear picture of what needs to happen and where to start. As you follow Jamie's example below, try filling out the visual organizer with a big project of your own:

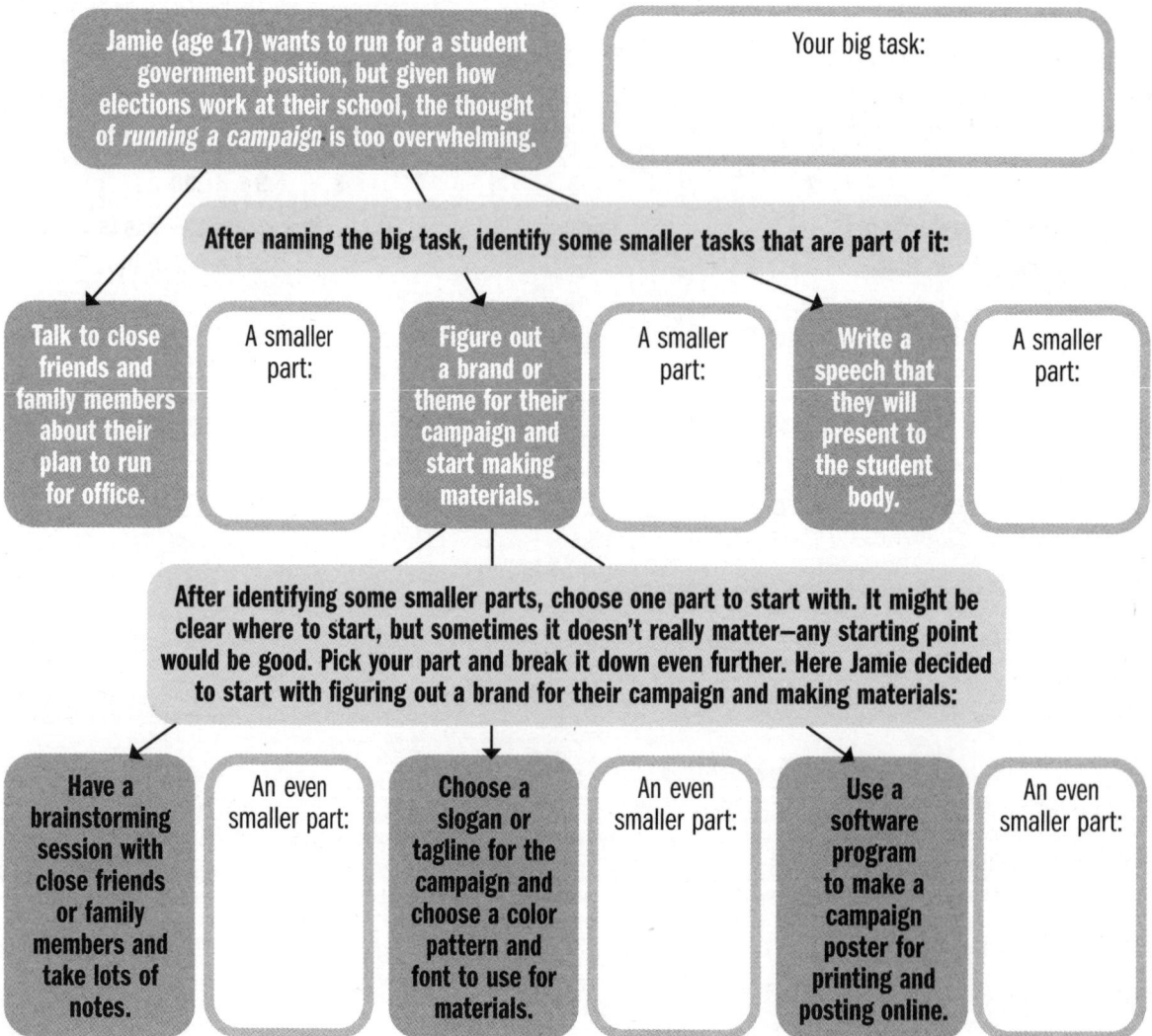

Jamie (age 17) wants to run for a student government position, but given how elections work at their school, the thought of *running a campaign* is too overwhelming.

Your big task:

After naming the big task, identify some smaller tasks that are part of it:

Talk to close friends and family members about their plan to run for office.

A smaller part:

Figure out a brand or theme for their campaign and start making materials.

A smaller part:

Write a speech that they will present to the student body.

A smaller part:

After identifying some smaller parts, choose one part to start with. It might be clear where to start, but sometimes it doesn't really matter—any starting point would be good. Pick your part and break it down even further. Here Jamie decided to start with figuring out a brand for their campaign and making materials:

Have a brainstorming session with close friends or family members and take lots of notes.

An even smaller part:

Choose a slogan or tagline for the campaign and choose a color pattern and font to use for materials.

An even smaller part:

Use a software program to make a campaign poster for printing and posting online.

An even smaller part:

Practice Playlists

Music can have a big impact on the way we feel our feelings. For this activity, spend some time making playlists for different situations that call for motivation. After completing this activity, you can actually make these playlists for the next time you need a boost. Share them on your favorite music platform so they might give others a boost too!

"Whenever I hear 'Shake It Off' by Taylor Swift, it gives me a boost of energy. I feel like I can handle any setback, and like things are going to turn out OK for me, if I just keep going."
—LEO, AGE 12

"It's an old song, but I love listening to 'Everybody Plays the Fool' by The Main Ingredient, especially when I'm recovering from a setback or a disappointment. It reminds me that not everything is going to go my way—and I can handle that." —SAORI, AGE 15

Songs that make me feel energetic and like I can do hard things:

Songs that help me keep going when I am in a good work groove:

Songs that I like to listen to when I am feeling sad or down and not very motivated:

Songs that make me feel like celebrating after I have done something important:

Knowing When to Quit

In our culture, stories about perseverance and **grit** are often celebrated, and most people would agree that these are important qualities. However, a **"don't be a quitter"** mentality assumes that we have unlimited time and energy. Unfortunately, that just isn't true—for anyone. Knowing when to stop and knowing when to keep going are important life skills, because they help us make good decisions about how to use the time and energy we do have. We also can learn a lot from our past experiences. Think about the following situations and illustrate or write about a time you experienced each one:

"I played on my school's junior varsity tennis team for two seasons because my parents told me that I needed to be 'well balanced' for my college applications. But there's no way any college would have been interested in my mediocre tennis-playing abilities. I wish I hadn't bothered with tennis at all and that I could have used that time to invest in the activities that I am actually good at and enjoy."
—JACOB, AGE 16

A time when you felt like quitting but kept going—and it was awesome:	A time when you felt like quitting but kept going—and maybe quitting would have worked out better:
A time when you felt like quitting and DID quit but regretted it later:	**A time when you felt like quitting and DID quit—and it turned out great:**

Taking Stock of My Activities

We often stick with the same activities, even if they're no longer fun or rewarding, just because we have been doing them for a long time and they're pretty much a habit. The beginning of the school year—or really anytime you find that you're not feeling satisfied with your activities—is a good time to take stock of your activities. In the worksheet below, write the different activities that you participate in, then rate your aptitude, pleasure, and practice for each one.

> "I had been taking dance classes since I was really little, but I didn't really enjoy them, and I always felt happy whenever class was canceled. I kept with it because I'd been doing it for so long and I thought it was really important to my mom. However, we had a long talk before I started high school. She understood that I wanted more time to devote to theater, and she was completely fine with me stopping dance lessons. I'm happier now, and I kind of wish we'd talked about it sooner." —JOLENE, AGE 15

Current activity (fill in each one)	Aptitude rating (circle/highlight one)	Pleasure rating (circle/highlight one)	Practice rating (circle/highlight one)
	3—I am great at this! 2—I'm decent. 1—I'm not so good.	3—Love it! 2—Like it. 1—Actively dislike it.	3—I do it all the time! 2—I do it quite a bit. 1—I don't do it much.
	3—I am great at this! 2—I'm decent. 1—I'm not so good.	3—Love it! 2—Like it. 1—Actively dislike it.	3—I do it all the time! 2—I do it quite a bit. 1—I don't do it much.
	3—I am great at this! 2—I'm decent. 1—I'm not so good.	3—Love it! 2—Like it. 1—Actively dislike it.	3—I do it all the time! 2—I do it quite a bit. 1—I don't do it much.
	3—I am great at this! 2—I'm decent. 1—I'm not so good.	3—Love it! 2—Like it. 1—Actively dislike it.	3—I do it all the time! 2—I do it quite a bit. 1—I don't do it much.
	3—I am great at this! 2—I'm decent. 1—I'm not so good.	3—Love it! 2—Like it. 1—Actively dislike it.	3—I do it all the time! 2—I do it quite a bit. 1—I don't do it much.
	3—I am great at this! 2—I'm decent. 1—I'm not so good.	3—Love it! 2—Like it. 1—Actively dislike it.	3—I do it all the time! 2—I do it quite a bit. 1—I don't do it much.
	3—I am great at this! 2—I'm decent. 1—I'm not so good.	3—Love it! 2—Like it. 1—Actively dislike it.	3—I do it all the time! 2—I do it quite a bit. 1—I don't do it much.

Pruning My Activity Tree

It probably sounds pretty obvious, but one of our main goals is to help you figure out and invest in the activities that you are good at, like doing, and do as often as you can. However, many of us still like to do things even when they do not come naturally to us and we have to work hard at them. Also, you might find that you have aptitudes in certain areas that don't actually bring you much pleasure. This is all normal and OK.

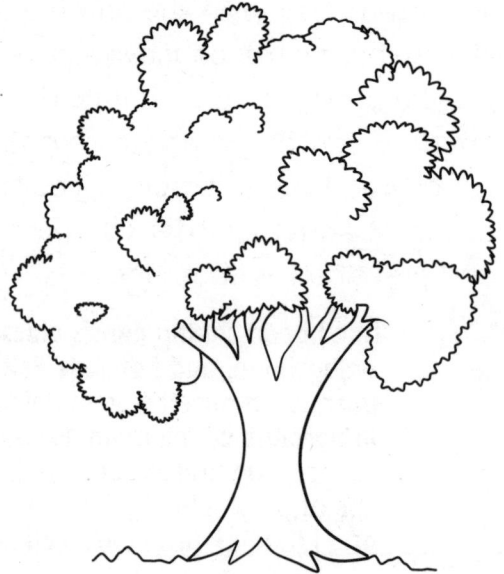

Knowing which activities you do not enjoy and find yourself avoiding is useful information—maybe just as helpful as knowing what you *do* like. Look back at your ratings on "Taking Stock of My Activities" (page 87). Did you have any 1s? Find the activity with the lowest rating and write it below. The following questions can help you decide whether to keep going with the activity or to prune your activity tree and spend your time doing something more motivating.

Activity with your lowest rating: _____

Why do you do this activity?

What would be good about ending this activity?

What would be hard about ending this activity?

If you ended this activity, what would you do with the time you currently spend on it?

Remember, ending an activity—even one you don't like—can be hard to do, because complicated factors are often involved. You can use this worksheet to help you decide what to do and then share it with your family.

"Through elementary school and middle school, I took private flute lessons in addition to playing in the school band. The summer before starting high school, I talked with my dad about continuing to play in the band, which is fun for me, but stopping private lessons, which are a lot less fun for me. I was nervous to talk with him about it because I thought he'd be disappointed, but he ended up being supportive."
—KAI, AGE 15

Turning Pleasure into Practice

"I had a lot of fun the few times I went rock-climbing, but it is hard for me to get to the rock-climbing gym." —SASHA, AGE 16

"I like studying in a quiet room at the library in my town, but I usually just end up studying at home." —HAILEY, AGE 14

Most people have some activities that they enjoy doing. However, there are lots of reasons why people—especially busy students—might not get to do these things as often as they would like (or at all). **What are some activities that you really enjoy but do not get to do as often as you would like?** Try to name three:

1. _____

2. _____

3. _____

What gets in the way of having time to do these activities?

Can you think of any changes that you could make so that you could do them more often?

Setbacks Happen

A normal part of setting goals, making changes, and doing things differently is running into **setbacks.** Setbacks can look a lot of different ways. For instance, an injury might prevent you from starting a new physical activity, like rock climbing, that you were excited to try. Another setback could be trying a new activity but, in doing so, realizing that you don't like it as much as you thought you would. It's important to recognize setbacks when they happen and to get around them the best you can so that you can get back to doing more of the things that make you happy.

Think of a time when things did not turn out the way you'd planned and you faced a setback. Write about or illustrate it here:

How did you know you were dealing with a setback?

"I knew I was dealing with a setback when my poems and stories weren't getting published in the school magazine, and I felt very sad about it."
—TAJ, AGE 14

Is this a setback you are still dealing with? If so, write about what you've done—if anything—to try to change it. If you've already figured out how to solve the setback, describe what you did here:

"I read the items that had been selected for the magazine, to try to understand what they were looking for. I also asked the editor for advice."
—TAJ, AGE 14

91

Getting Around Setbacks

Setbacks can be many things—disappointing, angering, frustrating, defeating, embarrassing, even devastating—but one thing they do not have to be is permanent. As you will explore in this activity, there are any number of ways to move around any setback. As you follow along with Sloane's setback, think about a setback you might be facing right now. Write down your ideas in the boxes below:

Step 1: Name the setback.

"I said that I wanted to start playing my guitar again, but I haven't touched it in ages."
—SLOANE, AGE 16

Your setback:

Step 2: Name the goal you are trying to reach.

"I want to play my guitar at least every other day, so three or four times per week."

Your goal:

Step 3: Think about some options for getting around your setback. Could you adjust your goal? Your actions? Or maybe both?

"I could adjust my goal to make it more reachable. I could block off time for playing in my planner."

Your options:

Step 4: Pick an option from Step 3 and try it out. See what happens!

"It's OK to start smaller. My revised goal is to play my guitar once this week for 15 minutes. I am going to block off time to do this in my planner."

Your choice:

Step 5: Think about how things went when you put your choice from Step 4 into practice. Did it work out? If so, nice job! If it didn't work, go back to your options from Step 3 and choose another one to try.

"It worked! Writing down my intention to practice guitar in my planner made it easier to do. I actually ended up playing twice!"

Your results:

Where Is My Practice Right Now?

In this chapter you completed many activities to help you think about how you spend your time and how you would *like* to be spending your time. Based on what you've learned about yourself and the things you spend your time doing, fill in the lines below.

Aptitude

Pleasure

Practice

Activities that I like to spend my time doing:

_____

_____

_____

_____

_____

_____

_____

_____

_____

_____

5

Pulling It All Together

Chapter 5 is about setting goals. Most activities ask kids to pull together information from other parts of the book so they can turn ideas into action plans. But this chapter isn't only about how to set good goals. It also gives kids the opportunity to learn about the differences between a fixed mindset and a growth mindset. It teaches kids ways to convey what they need from the adults in their lives so the adults can be fuel for motivation instead of motivation "killers."

Kids, especially kids who struggle with motivation, often have difficulty identifying the end game. Parents often think happiness is the end goal, but it's important to remember that happiness isn't a goal. It's the *result* of good goals. It's an outcome rather than the goal itself. Keep that in mind as you work through these activities with the child in your life. Identifying appropriate goals and using them to motivate behavior and find meaning in life is one of the most important ways to help your child. Because the activities in this chapter ask kids to pull together information from other chapters of the book, it's recommended to complete at least a couple of activities in each of the other chapters before starting this one.

Pulling It All Together

By this point, you have done a lot of reflecting on the things you are good at, the things you enjoy doing, and the things you spend your time doing. The overlap of these things is where your strongest motivation lives. Look back at the activities you've completed to fill in the diagram below:

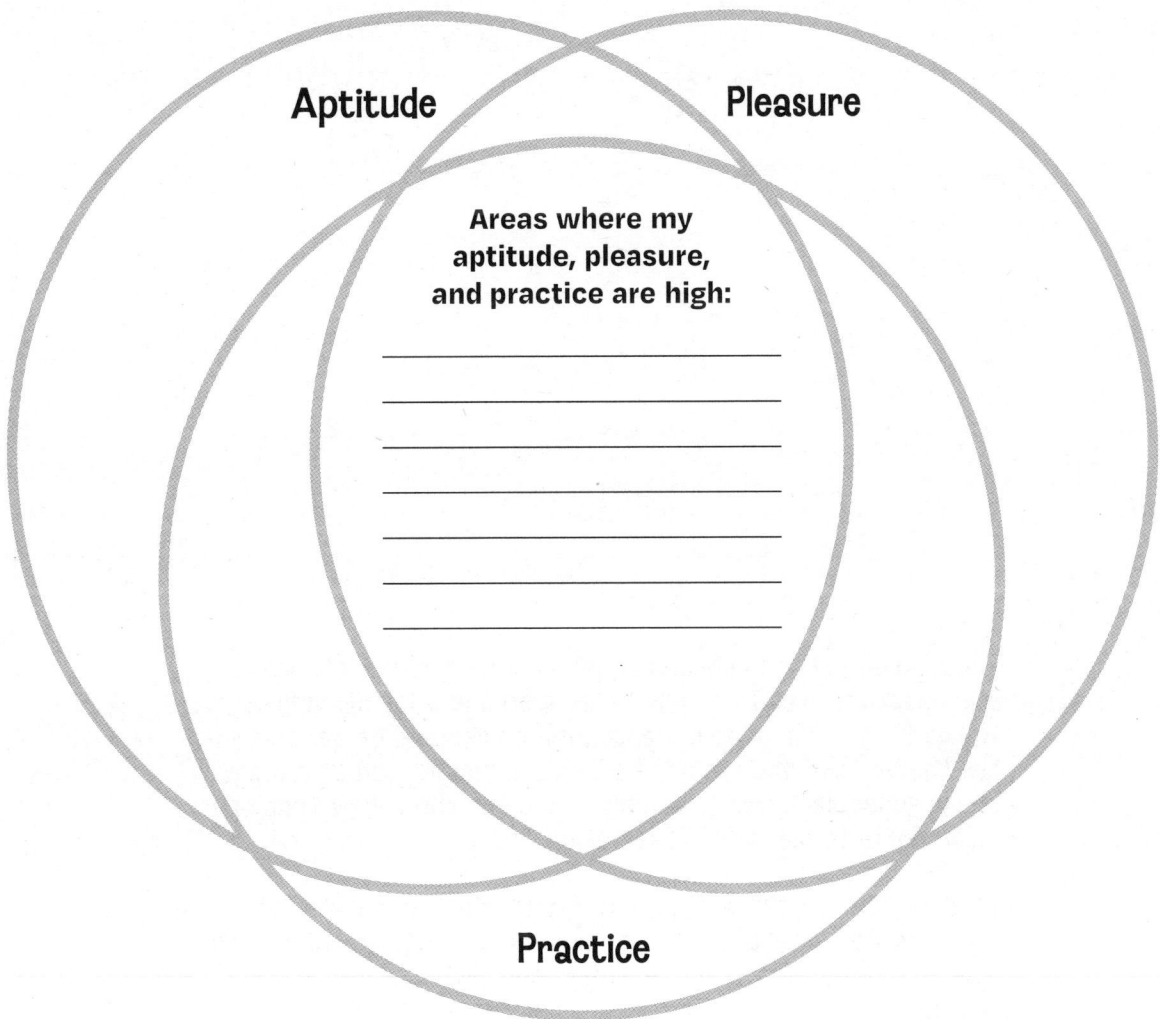

Aptitude　　　　　**Pleasure**

Areas where my aptitude, pleasure, and practice are high:

_____
_____
_____
_____
_____
_____
_____

Practice

Look back at the Venn diagram you completed at the beginning of this book (page 18). Compare what you completed then with what you just filled in.

What looks similar? What looks different? Take a moment to reflect on what you have learned about yourself by working through these activities, then write about it here:

"Once I stopped and really thought about aptitude, pleasure, and practice, I realized that I was spending a lot of time on things that other people wanted me to like and be good at—not the things I like and am good at. After making some changes to my schedule, I now have more time for the things that are meaningful to me, and it feels good."

—ADRIAN, AGE 14

"Thinking about aptitude, pleasure, and practice helped me realize that I do not have to spend my time only doing the things I am good at. Some things, like building Lego sets, are just for fun, and this works for me."

—WILLOW, AGE 12

"By trying some new activities, like pickleball, I realized that I have some strengths that I didn't even know about! Now that I do know about them, I make time for them."

—ZAC, AGE 15

Setting Good Goals

Setting goals is important—but not just *any* goals. How you set up goals for yourself plays an important role in how you work toward them. For over 40 years people across many different fields—business, technology, psychology, human resources, and more—have been setting something called SMART goals, and they can help you too. SMART is an acronym that reflects five important qualities that good goals have:

S = Specific (a narrow or specific goal is easier to work toward than a broad or vague one)

M = Measurable (you need ways to use numbers to track your progress toward your goal)

A = Achievable (to be meaningful, the goals you set need to be within your reach)

R = Relevant (your goals should make sense for you and line up with your bigger picture)

T = Time-limited (all good things need to come to an end—including your goals)

For this activity, let's revisit Sloane from "Getting Around Setbacks" (pages 92–93). She was having trouble in her attempt to play her guitar more often. Here we break down what a SMART goal for Sloane might look like. As you follow along with her goal, try developing a SMART goal of your own.

Sloane's original goal:

"I said that I wanted to start playing my guitar again, but I haven't touched it in ages."
—SLOANE, AGE 16

Your original goal:

Make it **specific:**

"I am going to choose one song to practice, prepare, and play at my school's talent show."

How can you make yours **specific?**

Make it **measurable:**

"I am going to practice for at least 15 minutes at a time, four times per week."

How can you make yours **measurable?**

Make it **attainable:**

"Since I am now getting back into playing guitar after a break, I am going to choose a song that I like and that will be pretty easy to learn."

How can you make yours **attainable?**

Make it **relevant:**

"Performing in an upcoming talent show feels like a great reason to start playing guitar again."

How can you make yours **relevant?**

Make it **time-limited:**

"The talent show is 6 weeks away. After I prepare and perform in the show, I will figure out a new guitar goal."

How can you make yours **time-limited?**

Pull it all together and name the **SMART goal:**

"My goal is to choose a fun, easy-to-learn song to play on my guitar, so that I can have fun and perform well in my school's talent show. I will practice the song I choose for at least 15 minutes, 4 days per week, for the next 6 weeks leading up to the talent show."

What is your new SMART goal?

Clearing My Path

By completing the different activities in this workbook, you likely have learned a lot about yourself. You can use this information toward making changes that will boost your motivation. Not all changes have to be big or difficult to make—sometimes the smallest tweaks and changes have the biggest impact.

Can you think of any small tweaks or changes that you could make to your environment right now? Think of this as **clearing your path** toward having greater motivation for all the things you need and want to do. Write your ideas for small changes in the empty boxes below:

"I am going to set up and decorate a space in my room for homework."
—CLEMENTINE, AGE 13

"I am going to talk to my parents about feeling overscheduled."
—NATHAN, AGE 16

Fixed Mindset versus Growth Mindset

You may already be familiar with the concepts of fixed mindset and growth mindset, or this might be new information for you. Basically, a **mindset** is a collection of ideas and beliefs that we hold about ourselves and our surroundings. In turn, these powerful thoughts shape our actions and our behaviors—and our actions and behaviors shape our mindset too.

People who have a **fixed mindset** believe "it is what it is." They often think that the way things are now is how they are always going to be. With this mindset, it can feel pointless to try to make positive changes or to do things differently. Folks with a fixed mindset ask, "What's the point?" It becomes easy to see how a fixed mindset goes hand in hand with low motivation.

It is normal to have a fixed mindset about some things and a growth mindset about others. Are there any areas of your life where you notice having a fixed mindset? Write some of the thoughts that are part of your fixed mindset in the bubbles below.

An area where my mindset is fixed: _____

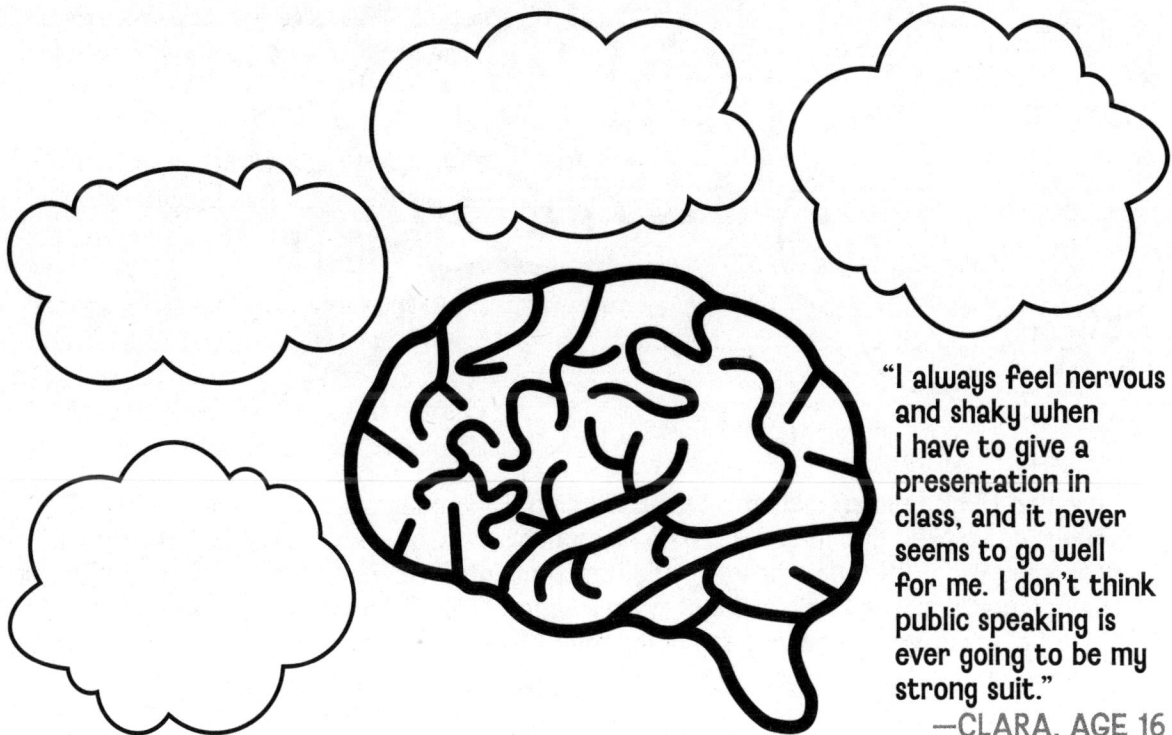

"I always feel nervous and shaky when I have to give a presentation in class, and it never seems to go well for me. I don't think public speaking is ever going to be my strong suit."
—CLARA, AGE 16

103

People who have a **growth mindset** think differently. They think there is always room for things to change, grow, and get better. The way things are right now is simply a starting point. Just as a fixed mindset is associated with low motivation, a growth mindset is associated with higher motivation.

Are there any areas of your life where you notice having a growth mindset? Think about whether your growth mindset is something you've always had or something you've had to develop along the way. Write some of the thoughts that are part of your growth mindset in the bubbles below.

An area where I have a growth mindset: _____

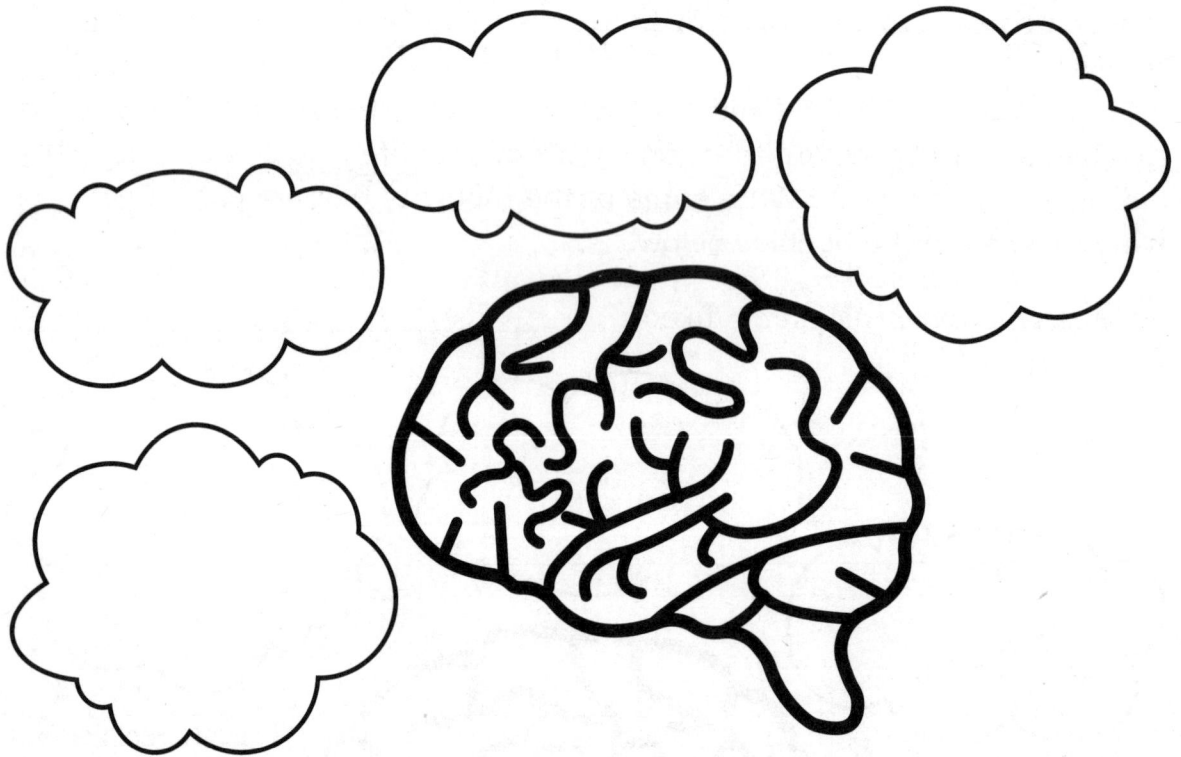

"I used to think I wasn't athletic because I didn't like competing in games and I always got picked last in gym class in elementary school. Once I started jogging and preparing for a 5K race, though, I realized that 'athletic' can mean a lot of different things. Just because I didn't like gym class when I was little doesn't mean that I can't enjoy being active and moving my body now."
—MIA, AGE 15

Goal Stories—Part I

Hearing stories about times that people set goals and worked hard to achieve them can feel inspiring and motivating. They also can contain helpful information that we can use as we go in search of our own goals. For this activity, interview an adult in your life about a time when they set and achieved an important goal. Ask them the following questions and think about their answers:

What is one important goal that you set for yourself and worked hard to achieve?

_____

_____

Why was this goal important to you?

_____

_____

How did you work toward this goal?

_____

_____

Did anything get in your way while you were working on your goal? If so, what did you do about it?

_____

_____

Looking back, would you have done anything differently?

_____

_____

What did you learn about yourself as a result of achieving your goal?

_____

_____

Goal Stories—Part II

We do not necessarily achieve each and every goal that we set for ourselves. As you will see, this is a normal part of setting and working toward goals. As much as we learn from the goals we do achieve, we sometimes learn even more from the ones we do not. For this activity, interview an adult in your life about a time they did NOT achieve a goal they had set out to do. Ask them the following questions and think about their answers:

What is one goal that you set for yourself but did not end up achieving?

_____

_____

Why was this goal important to you?

_____

_____

How did you work toward this goal?

_____

_____

What ended up getting in your way or otherwise made it not possible to achieve this goal?

_____

_____

Looking back, would you still have set the same goal for yourself? Or a different one?

_____

_____

What did you learn about yourself as a result of NOT achieving your goal?

_____

_____

Goal Stories—My Turn

Illustrate or write about a time that you set a goal for yourself—and you achieved it. What was the goal? How did you complete it? How did it feel? What did you learn?

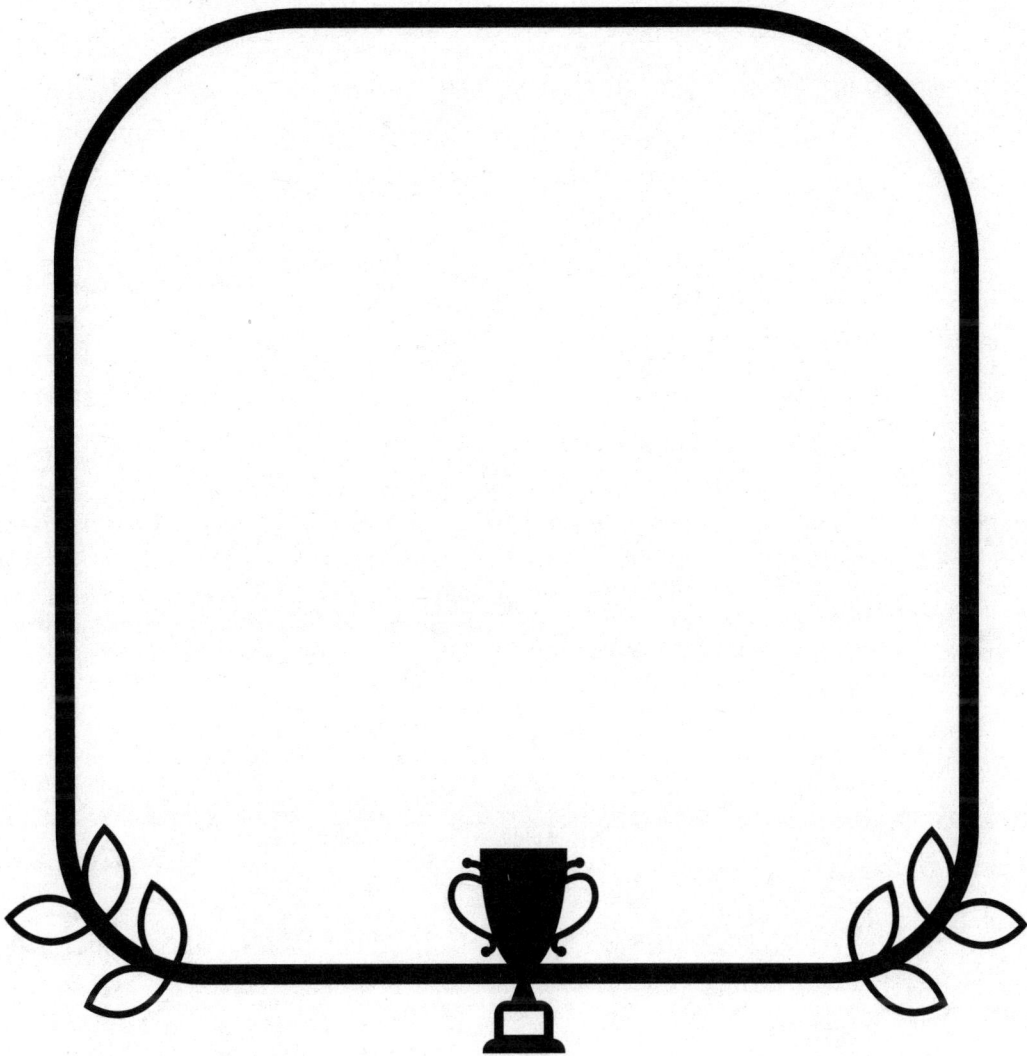

"I felt like I succeeded when I was chosen to be editor-in-chief of my high school's newspaper. I had been working toward it, and hoping for it, with every article I had written as a freshman and sophomore. It felt like a lot of responsibility, which made me feel nervous, but I also knew that I was prepared to take on the role. Even if it would feel uncomfortable at times, I knew I would learn a lot as I went along."
—DANI, AGE 16

Even when we do not achieve a goal that we set for ourselves, there can be a lot of helpful learning along the way. Illustrate or write about a time that you set a goal for yourself—and you didn't achieve it. What was the goal? What happened instead? How did it feel? What did you learn?

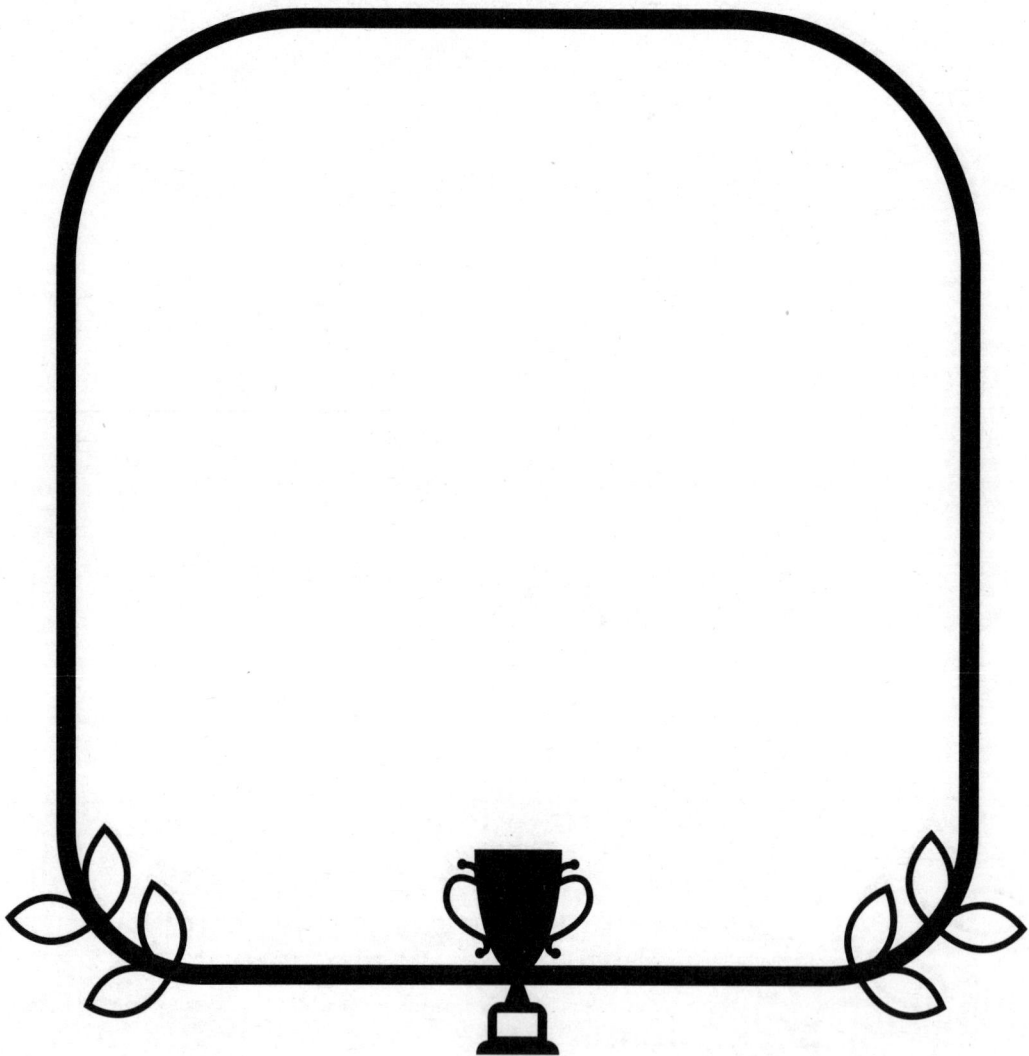

"I ran for class treasurer, but I did not get elected. I felt very disappointed and even a little embarrassed. However, I learned that it's okay to put myself out there and go after the things I want. It doesn't feel good, but I can handle it when things don't work out the way I want them to."
—CLARKE, AGE 14

More of This, Less of That—
Parent Version

Parents can say or do things to try to motivate their kids, but they end up missing the mark and having the opposite effect. Has this ever happened to you? Sometimes parents need guidance about how to be helpful and motivating. This activity helps you identify the **helpful** things your parents might say or do and the **unhelpful** things they might say or do.

Hint: Look back at your work on "Don't Marsh My Mellow!" on page 57 for ideas about what the adults in your life could be doing LESS of.

MORE of this . . .   **. . . and LESS of this**

"I don't mind going to weekend tutoring so much because my dad and I always get hot chocolate afterward." —TOMAS, AGE 13

"It isn't helpful when my mom threatens to ground me or take my phone away if I don't start my homework." —VIGGO, AGE 14

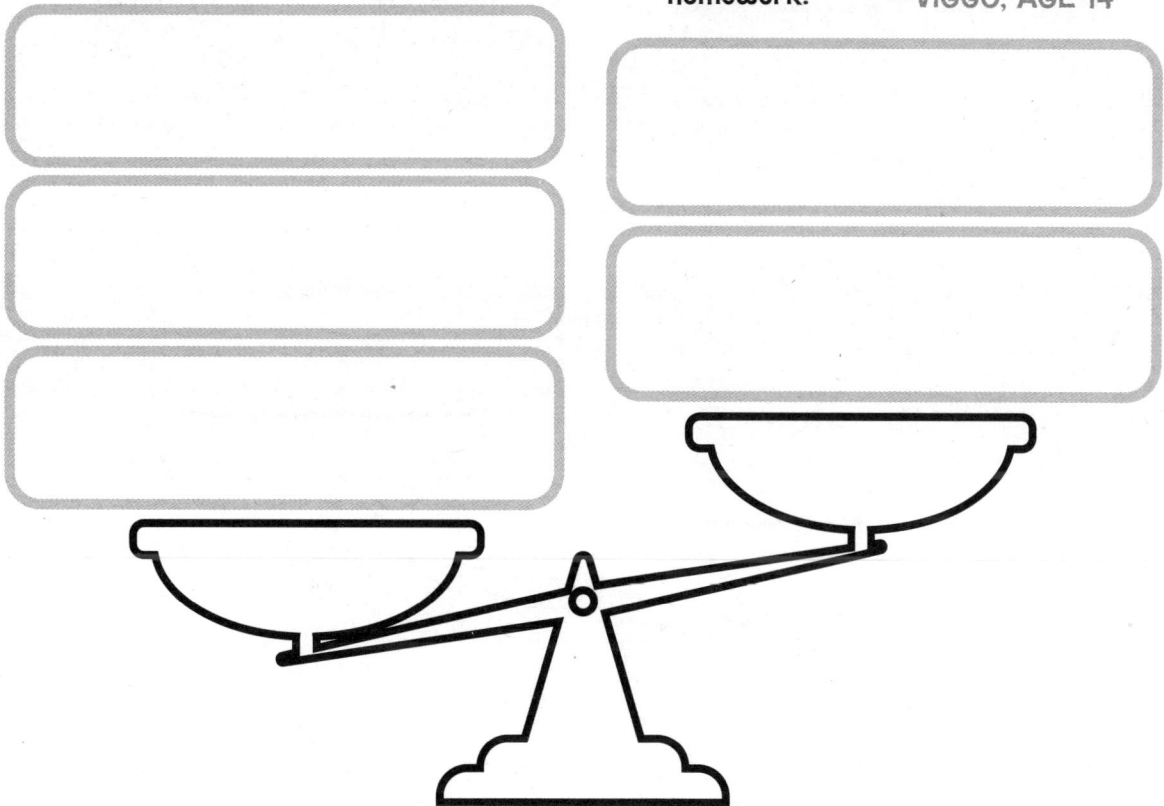

More of This, Less of That— Teacher and Coach Version

Just like parents, teachers and coaches can say or do things to try to be motivating but miss the mark and end up having the opposite effect. Teachers and coaches also need guidance about how to be helpful and motivating. This activity helps you identify the **helpful** things the teachers or coaches in your life might say or do and the **unhelpful** things they might say or do.

Hint: Look back at your work on "Don't Marsh My Mellow!" on page 57 for ideas about what the adults in your life could be doing **less** of.

MORE of this . . .   **. . . and LESS of this**

"It is helpful when teachers are really clear and direct with me and let me know when I am doing a good job." —MARIELA, AGE 12

"I don't like it when teachers make us have debates in class. Some students love it, but it just makes me nervous." —CAMERON, AGE 13

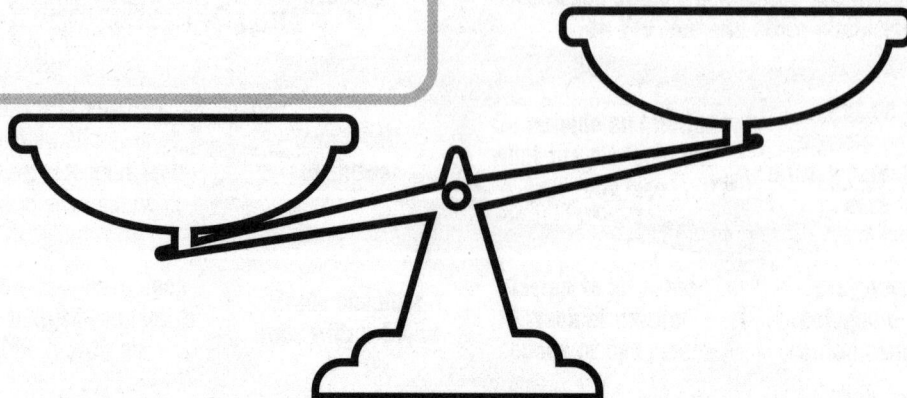

Adult Education

Look back at the ideas you came up with in the "More of This, Less of That" activities (pages 109–110). You have some valuable and insightful information—now you need to share it with the people who need it, the people who are rooting for you. The goal of this activity is to give the adults in your life the information they need to support you better.

The following are some ideas for sharing important information with the adults in your life. Color in or highlight the ones that you could see yourself doing.

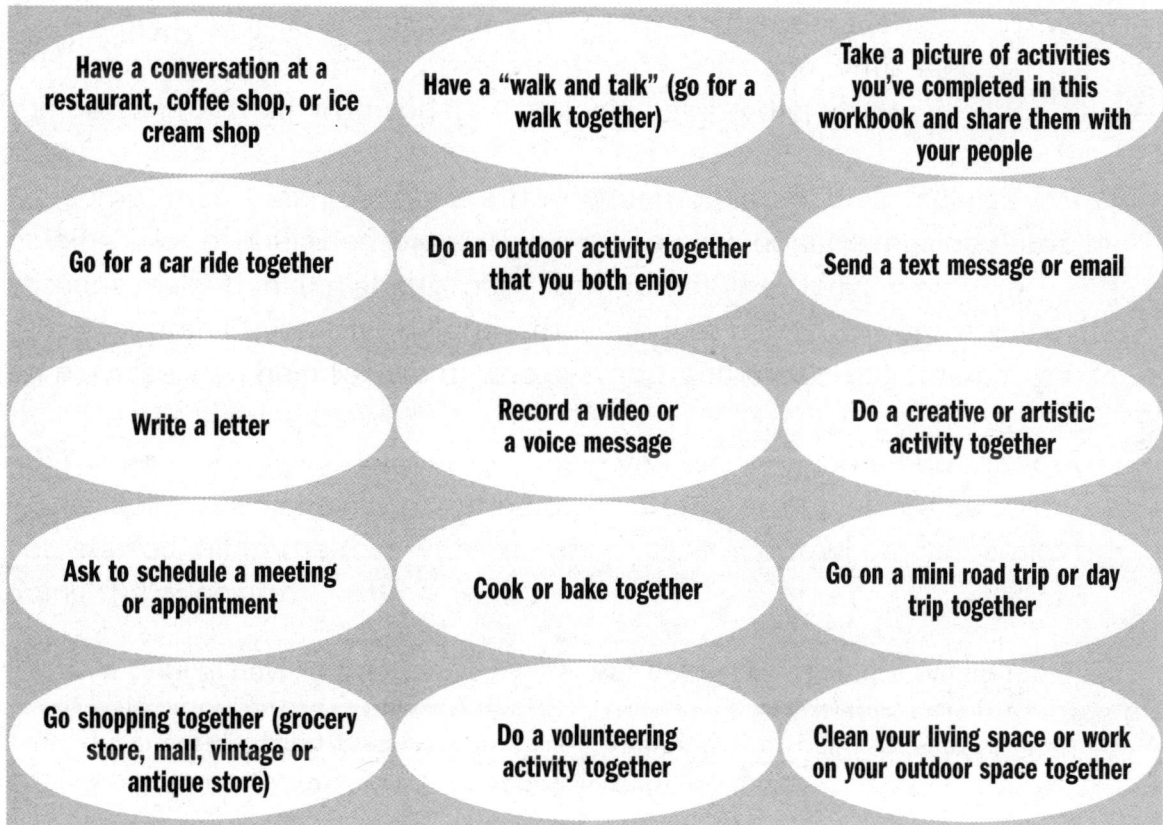

Have a conversation at a restaurant, coffee shop, or ice cream shop	Have a "walk and talk" (go for a walk together)	Take a picture of activities you've completed in this workbook and share them with your people
Go for a car ride together	Do an outdoor activity together that you both enjoy	Send a text message or email
Write a letter	Record a video or a voice message	Do a creative or artistic activity together
Ask to schedule a meeting or appointment	Cook or bake together	Go on a mini road trip or day trip together
Go shopping together (grocery store, mall, vintage or antique store)	Do a volunteering activity together	Clean your living space or work on your outdoor space together

A big hint: Use positive reinforcement to your advantage! Tell people when they are being helpful. You might find that they do it even more!

If this is something you'd like to do, but you're not sure how to put it into action, flip ahead to "Turning Ideas into Action Plans" on pages 112–113.

Turning Ideas into Action Plans

The activities in this workbook ask you to do a lot of thinking and reflecting. We know that this takes a lot of work. You also might like to try putting some of your good ideas into practice. Sometimes making changes can be pretty easy to do, but other times it can be really hard. Use these questions to take an idea and turn it into an action plan:

What is the thing you want to do or change? Try to be as clear as possible.

When and where are you going to do it?

Do you need transportation, special materials, or help from anyone else to do it? If so, what is your plan for getting these things in place?

Is your plan possible to put into place? Does anything about it need to be changed so that you are more likely to do it?

Is there anything that could get in your way? How might you get around any roadblocks?

How are you going to follow through with your plan and keep up your motivation?

How will you know when you have completed your plan?

How are you going to document or celebrate following through with your plan?

Feeling Proud of How I've Changed

Sometimes we find ourselves in situations that remind us of how far we have come and how much we have changed—for the better. After all, there is a reason why "how it started versus how it's going" is a cultural phenomenon. Can you think of a recent time you did something easily that would have been a challenge for you in the past? Write about or illustrate it below.

Hint: If you need some ideas to get started, look back at your work on "Double Meanings" (see page 40–41). Are there any areas where you have started turning a weakness into a strength?

How it started:

How it's going:

Example:
"Last year I put off writing history papers until the last minute, then stayed up all night to finish them. My papers never ended up being very good, and I always felt gross the next day."

Example:
"Last week, I felt proud of myself for starting early on my history project. I made an outline first. Once I jumped in and started writing, it was pretty easy to keep going."

"When something happens and it makes me feel like I've grown or changed a lot, it makes me feel really proud. I call it a 'goal post moment' because it reminds me of how far I've come from where I was before."
—OLIVIA, AGE 13

6

A Few Other Things That Can Get in the Way of Motivation

The previous chapters of this workbook have given you a fundamental understanding of motivation, as well as a new framework—consisting of aptitude, pleasure, and practice—for thinking about it. Very often, what looks like "low motivation" in a child or teen can be more helpfully understood as a "mismatch problem" among the things they are good at doing, they like doing, and they spend their time doing. This mismatch could be the result of their own decision making, though quite often it is the result of messaging from well-meaning adults in their lives. The earlier activities in this workbook were designed to help kids take an honest inventory of their aptitudes, pleasures, and practices and to help them share this newfound knowledge with the adults who care most about them. We continue to be optimistic, enthusiastic, and confident that these steps will help our young readers feel greater motivation in their day-to-day lives and build lives that they are excited to lead.

Still, there are factors beyond aptitude, pleasure, and practice that can impact one's motivation and zest for life, and that is what this final chapter is all about. The following activities tap into feelings of not caring (which is widely recognized as an aspect of burnout), sleep, movement, screen time, relaxation, and choosing intentional or "opposite" actions. These activities include psychoeducation, based in both research and our clinical experiences, that is likely to be helpful for any reader.

Signs and Signals of Not Caring

Imagine a trash can full of garbage. The garbage is all the things that keep you from feeling motivated and caring about things. In the trash can below, shade in or highlight where you think your garbage level is right now:

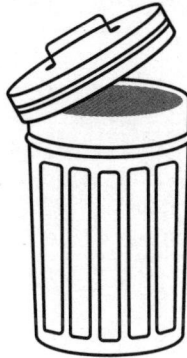

Overflowing

Pretty full

Getting fuller

Pretty low

Now think about the garbage in your trash can. Shade in or highlight the items that are filling up your trash can:

- Not feeling like doing anything
- Feeling anxious
- Feeling stuck
- Not getting enough or good-quality sleep
- Feeling irritable or easily angered
- Making plans but then canceling them
- Feeling sad
- Not wanting to try new things
- Feeling disorganized
- Avoiding responding to messages
- Worrying about my future
- Feeling bored
- Giving up easily, even when it's something I want to do
- Waiting until the last minute to start assignments
- Not doing the things I'm supposed to do
- Spending more time than I mean to on my phone or playing video games
- Feeling dumb (even when people say I'm smart)
- Not caring about what happens in the future

Many people find that the fuller their trash can is, the harder it is to take out. Do you currently have any go-to strategies for taking out the garbage in your trash can? If so, write them here:

"When I feel my trash can getting too full, I like to go outside and run down the sidewalk as fast as I possibly can. It helps."

—EMMY, AGE 12

Think about how well the strategies you wrote above are working (or not working). The goal of the activities in this chapter is to help you identify other things that are filling your trash can. They also help you come up with some new ideas for taking out your own trash can before it gets too full.

Sleeping Better

When you're not getting enough sleep, there are probably a lot of other things that are not going well either. Research shows us that sleep has many important benefits for physical health, mental health, attention, concentration, energy level, and—you guessed it—motivation. Sleep is the foundation for all other healthy functioning. Research also shows us that about 60% of middle schoolers and 70% of high schoolers report not getting enough sleep on school nights. If you find that your motivation level is chronically low, an important, early step is to take a good look at your sleep.

While many biological, behavioral, environmental, and cultural factors work together to impact sleep, there are fortunately many things within our control that can improve our sleep. Below are a lot of things that make up good sleep hygiene (healthy sleep habits) for teens. For each one, rate how it currently looks for you:

Getting the recommended amount of sleep (9–12 hours for kids 6–12 years old, 8–10 hours for teenagers)	☐ I rarely or never do this.	☐ This sometimes goes well for me.	☐ This looks great for me!
Keeping a consistent sleep schedule, including wake-up and bedtimes, on both school nights and weekends	☐ I rarely or never do this.	☐ This sometimes goes well for me.	☐ This looks great for me!
Following a consistent bedtime routine (bathing, brushing teeth, putting on pajamas) that cues your body that it'll be time to sleep soon	☐ I rarely or never do this.	☐ This sometimes goes well for me.	☐ This looks great for me!
Skipping drinks containing stimulants like caffeine, especially past morning hours	☐ I rarely or never do this.	☐ This sometimes goes well for me.	☐ This looks great for me!
Putting away your computer, phone, tablet, and other screen devices at least 30 minutes before going to bed	☐ I rarely or never do this.	☐ This sometimes goes well for me.	☐ This looks great for me!
Making sure your sleeping area is a cool, comfortable temperature	☐ I rarely or never do this.	☐ This sometimes goes well for me.	☐ This looks great for me!

Making sure your sleeping area is quiet (or has soft, gentle white or ambient noise, if this helps you sleep)	☐ I rarely or never do this.	☐ This sometimes goes well for me.	☐ This looks great for me!
Making sure your mattress, sheets, comforter, blanket, pillows, and any other bedding are all comfortable (and not too warm)	☐ I rarely or never do this.	☐ This sometimes goes well for me.	☐ This looks great for me!
Making sure your sleeping area is dark	☐ I rarely or never do this.	☐ This sometimes goes well for me.	☐ This looks great for me!
Exercising or moving your body during the day (but not too close to bedtime)	☐ I rarely or never do this.	☐ This sometimes goes well for me.	☐ This looks great for me!
Saving your bed only for sleep and moving all other activities (like reading, doing homework, using your phone) out of your bed	☐ I rarely or never do this.	☐ This sometimes goes well for me.	☐ This looks great for me!
Spending time outside every day	☐ I rarely or never do this.	☐ This sometimes goes well for me.	☐ This looks great for me!
Sticking to calm, quiet, and relaxing activities before bedtime (instead of activities that are likely to make you feel more awake)	☐ I rarely or never do this.	☐ This sometimes goes well for me.	☐ This looks great for me!
Getting out of bed to do a gentle activity if you haven't fallen asleep after around 20 minutes after getting into bed	☐ I rarely or never do this.	☐ This sometimes goes well for me.	☐ This looks great for me!

Look at your ratings above. Do you see any patterns? Take a moment now and think about one thing that you could try tonight (or at least soon) to get better sleep:

Moving More

Like sleep, physical activity and movement are known to have important benefits for mental and physical health. If you find that your motivation level is low, looking closely at your activity level is an important early step too. According to the U.S. Centers for Disease Control and Prevention (CDC), children and teens should have 1 hour of physical activity daily. Of course, this is a general recommendation—before changing your activity level, it is important to talk to your parents and doctor about your own situation and activity needs.

Below are some common—and less common—ways of increasing movement in your daily activities. Shade in or highlight the ones that you could picture yourself trying soon.

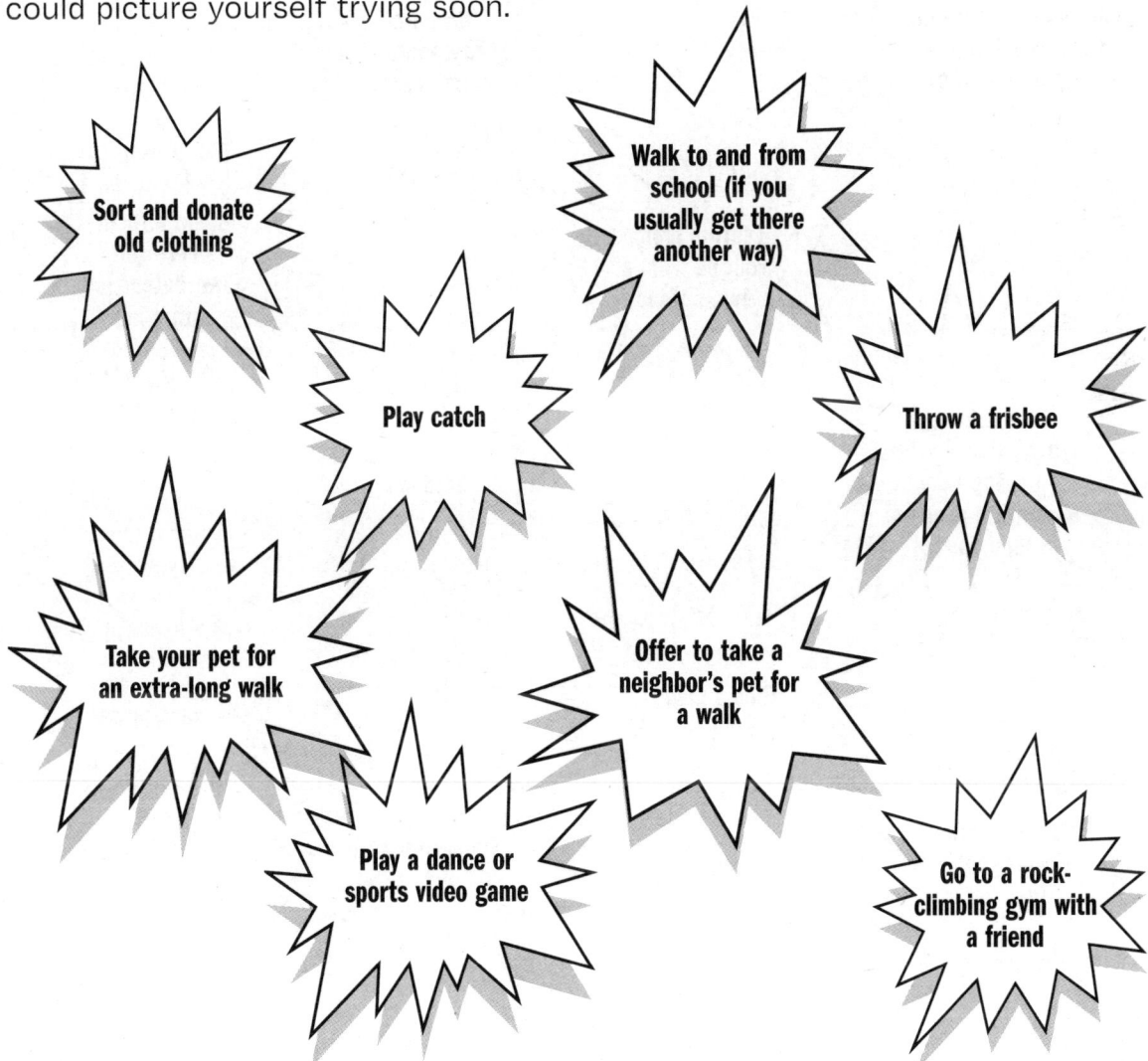

Sort and donate old clothing

Walk to and from school (if you usually get there another way)

Play catch

Throw a frisbee

Take your pet for an extra-long walk

Offer to take a neighbor's pet for a walk

Play a dance or sports video game

Go to a rock-climbing gym with a friend

Do yoga poses

Stretch

Play a physical game (like tag, Twister)

Play with younger siblings or relatives

Stand, walk, or move around during activities where you'd usually be sitting

Have an impromptu dance party

Learn a dance routine from a music video

Clean a room where you live (kitchen, bathroom)

Do a volunteer activity that involves moving (like organizing goods at a food pantry)

Garden

Ride a bike

Sit on an exercise ball

Run an errand for a family member

Do your homework at a standing desk

Screen Time Activity

Most kids enjoy using their phones, tablets, computers, and other devices, **and** they want to change their habits. This activity can help you have a different kind of relationship with your devices.

Phones and tablets have built-in tracking software that can give you helpful information about your overall usage habits, as well as the apps you use most often and how much time you spend on them. This information alone, however, might not give you everything you need to understand **why** you use your devices and how to start making changes.

If you want to change the way you use your devices, we encourage you to start by collecting some data about your current patterns. This worksheet helps you think about your screen usage as a **behavior** that serves a purpose. Try using this worksheet to track the way you use technology over the course of one day:

Day and time screen time started/total time spent	How did you spend your screen time?	What was going on before screen time started?	What happened after screen time ended?	How did this screen time make you feel?
Monday, 7:00 p.m. 45 minutes	Watching short videos on TikTok	I was about to start doing my math homework.	I went to the bathroom and got a snack before finally starting my homework.	It was kind of fun, but I was worried about my homework at the same time. I felt even more "meh" about it after screen time.

Do you see any patterns or surprises in your responses? Write about what you noticed here:

Below are some ideas for using screen time less or differently. Shade in or highlight the ones you could see yourself trying soon.

Turn off your phone for 24 hours and see what you notice

Try using an app that limits your access to certain websites and/or total amount of screen time per day

Try using a low-tech method or version of something you'd normally use your phone for (like a paper to-do list, stopwatch, book)

Treat screen time as a reward that you have to earn (like completing all homework before using your phone)

Tell other people about your plan to use screen time less

Swap time you'd normally spend on your phone with other fun activities (like playing a board game, doing a craft project)

Take a moment now to think about one thing you could try today (or at least soon) to start changing your relationship with screen time and your devices:

"It was painful at first, but ultimately it was helpful when I started giving my phone to my parents right before I started my homework. Without checking my phone all the time, I was able to get my work done quite a bit faster. And I didn't feel so bad about using my phone once I had finished my work." —AMELIA, AGE 16

Relaxing Better

"When I feel relaxed, I notice how my chest moves when I'm breathing evenly."
—CHLOE, AGE 14

Take a moment and think about what it feels like in your body when you are very relaxed. Color in or highlight the areas where you feel it here:

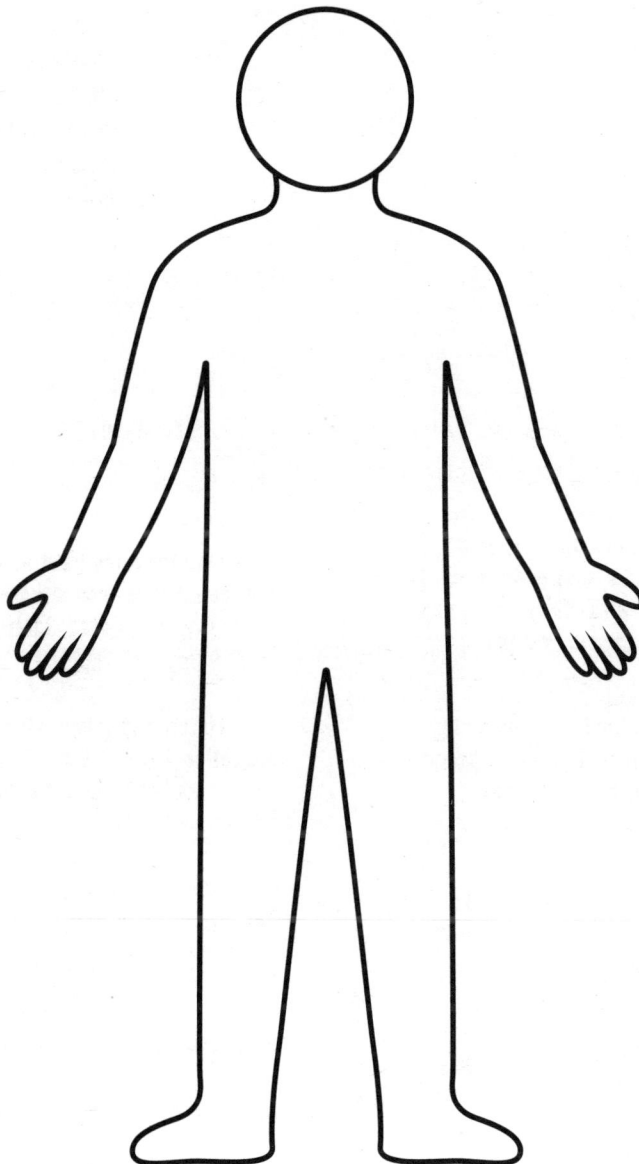

Most people find that relaxation feels really good. Fortunately, there are ways we can help our bodies feel more relaxed. Even better, giving ourselves relaxed feelings doesn't have to require any special or fancy equipment or cost any money. It doesn't even require much time! Think about relaxation as a muscle. The more you practice **applied relaxation** skills, the stronger, faster, and easier they will become.

What are some strategies you already have for helping yourself feel relaxed? Illustrate or write about them here:

"I have a set of different scented lotions that my grandmother once gave me. Smelling each of them deeply makes me feel relaxed."

—PAIGE, AGE 13

Below are different types of applied relaxation strategies. Shade in or highlight the ones you could see yourself trying soon:

- Listen and follow along with a progressive muscle relaxation audio track (which will guide you through tensing and relaxing different muscle groups)
- Pause for a moment and pay attention to what you notice through each of your five senses (sight, hearing, taste, touch, smell)
- Close your eyes and imagine being in a place in nature that you find peaceful (like the beach or woods)
- Listen and follow along with a guided meditation audio track (these are widely available on YouTube and other platforms)
- Squeeze a stress ball, Play-Doh, slime, or something else that feels good in your hands
- Take a bath or shower
- Go outside and notice what the air feels like on your face
- Put on fuzzy slippers or walk on a fuzzy carpet with your bare feet
- Take slow and even, deep breaths that fill your lungs and belly with air
- Trade shoulder rubs with a friend
- Listen to an audio track of nature sounds or spa music
- Spray perfume or cologne or sniff a scented candle deeply

Opposite Day

Changing our usual routines and activities is often easier said than done. One common way of making changes easier to attempt is to start by making small ones and do just a little bit at a time. In fact, this is the spirit of a lot of the activities in this chapter. We are firm believers that, indeed, a little can go a long way. And, as they say, a journey of a thousand miles begins with a single step.

At the same time, there are other ways that good, meaningful change can happen. One of those ways is by choosing **on purpose** to do the opposite thing from what we'd typically do. When you were younger, did your school ever have "Opposite Day"? This is where students might wear their clothing backward and socks on their hands and write their names at the bottom of their worksheets. The logic behind this strategy is kind of like that!

Sometimes, when people are feeling unmotivated, their feelings end up guiding a lot of their behaviors. This can look like doing things on autopilot, without really thinking about them. Sometimes the things we do on autopilot aren't even that helpful—they are just habits. Doing the opposite, on purpose, can help "shake up the system" and break up some patterns that are not serving us well.

The goal of this worksheet is to help you identify some current activities where doing the opposite might help you. Some examples are below to get you started; fill in the rest with your own ideas about where you could try doing the opposite:

On a typical day, I'd usually . . .	But doing the opposite would look like . . .
Hit the snooze button three or four times before finally getting out of bed	Jumping out of bed as soon as my alarm went off

On a typical day, I'd usually . . . **But doing the opposite would look like . . .**

On a typical day, I'd usually . . .	But doing the opposite would look like . . .
Doomscroll on social media for a while before starting my homework	Leaving my phone in the kitchen while I go upstairs to do my homework

Resources

There are many great sources of more information on topics covered in this book. Here are a few of the best. All of the books can be accessed through your public library, and the websites are free to the public. We've broken these down into resources for kids and those that are appropriate for the adults in their lives.

Resources for Kids and Teens

Books

Eidens, A. (2018). *Big Life Journal: Teen Edition.* Stamford, CT: Eidens.

Lohmann, R. C. (2019). *The Anger Workbook for Teens.* Oakland, CA: New Harbinger.

Sedley, B. (2017). *Stuff that Sucks: A Teen's Guide to Accepting What You Can't Change and Committing to What You Can.* Oakland, CA: New Harbinger.

Tompkins, M. A. (2020). *Zero to 60: A Teen's Guide to Manage Frustration, Anger, and Everyday Irritations.* Washington, DC: Magination Press.

Tompkins, M. A. (2023). *Stress Less: A Teen's Guide to a Calm Chill Life.* Washington, DC: Magination Press.

Tompkins, M. A., & Thompson, M. A. (2019). *The Insomnia Workbook for Teens.* Oakland, CA: New Harbinger.

Zucker, B. (2022). *A Perfectionist's Guide to Not Being Perfect.* Washington, DC: Magination Press.

Websites

The Clay Center for Young Healthy Minds: *www.mghclaycenter.org*
Nemours KidsHealth: *www.kidshealth.org/en/kids*
Nemours TeensHealth: *www.kidshealth.org/en/teens*
WOOP: *www.woopmylife.org/en/home*

Mobile Apps

Breathe2Relax
Happier Meditation: *www.meditatehappier.com*
Happy Not Perfect: Meditation and Mindfulness
Headspace
Healthy Minds Program: *www.hminnovations.org/meditation-app*
The Mindfulness App: *www.themindfulnessapp.com*
Three Good Things: A Happiness Journal: *www.the3goodthings.org/about*

Podcasts

Mostly Mindful for Teens and Tweens
This Teenage Life

Resources for Parents, Teachers, and Caregivers

Books

Clear, J. (2018). *Atomic Habits: An Easy and Proven Way to Build Good Habits and Break Bad Ones.* London, UK: Penguin.
Damour, L. (2023). *The Emotional Lives of Teenagers: Raising Connected, Capable, and Compassionate Adolescents.* New York: Ballantine.
Delman, M. (2018). *Your Kid's Gonna Be Okay: A Guide to Raising Competent and Confident Kids.* Needham, MA: Beyond Booksmart.
Dweck, C. S. (2016). *Mindset: The New Psychology of Success.* New York: Random House.
Fagell, P. L. (2023). *Middle School Superpowers: Raising Resilient Tweens in Turbulent Times.* New York: Hachette.
Gold, J. (2015). *Screen-Smart Parenting: How to Find Balance and Benefit in*

Your Child's Use of Social Media, Apps, and Digital Devices. New York: Guilford Press.

Hibbs, B. J., & Rostain, A. (2019). *The Stressed Years of Their Lives: Helping Your Child Survive and Thrive during Their College Years.* New York: St. Martin's Press.

Icard, M. (2024). *Eight Setbacks That Can Make a Child a Success.* New York: Rodale Books.

Lahey, J. (2015). *The Gift of Failure: How the Best Parents Learn to Let Go So Their Children Can Succeed.* New York: Harper Collins.

Levine, M. (2021). *Ready or Not: Preparing Our Kids to Thrive in an Uncertain and Rapidly Changing World.* New York: HarperCollins.

Lythcott-Haims, J. (2015). *How to Raise an Adult: Break Free of the Overparenting Trap and Prepare Your Kid for Success.* New York: Henry Holt and Co.

McCready, A. (2016). *The Me, Me, Me Epidemic: A Step-by-Step Guide to Raising Capable, Grateful Kids in an Over-Entitled World.* New York: TarcherPerigee.

Nelson, M. K. (2012). *Parenting Out of Control: Anxious Parents in Uncertain Times.* New York: New York University Press.

Payne, K. J., & Ross, L. M. (2020). *Simplicity Parenting.* New York: Ballantine Books.

Pressman, A. (2024). *The Five Principles of Parenting.* New York: Simon and Schuster.

Siegel, D. J., & Bryson, T. P. (2012). *The Whole-Brain Child: 12 Revolutionary Strategies to Nurture Your Child's Developing Mind* (Illustrated ed.). New York: Bantam.

Stixrud, W., & Johnson, N. (2019). *The Self-Driven Child: The Science and Sense of Giving Your Kids More Control over Their Lives.* London, UK: Penguin.

Stixrud, W., & Johnson, N. (2021). *What Do You Say?: How to Talk with Kids to Build Motivation, Stress Tolerance, and a Happy Home.* New York: Viking.

Wallace, J. B. (2023). *Never Enough: When Achievement Culture Becomes Toxic—And What We Can Do About It.* New York: Portfolio.

Waters, L. (2017). *The Strength Switch: How The New Science of Strength-Based Parenting Can Help Your Child and Your Teen to Flourish.* New York: Avery.

Weissbourd, R. (2010). *The Parents We Mean to Be: How Well-Intentioned Adults Undermine Children's Moral and Emotional Development.* Boston: Houghton Mifflin Harcourt.

Websites

American Academy of Pediatrics: Family Media Plan: *www.healthychildren. org/English/fmp/Pages/MediaPlan.aspx*

Fatherly: *www.fatherly.com*

Growth Mindset Institute: *www.growthmindsetinstitute.org*

Lisa Damour, PhD: *www.drlisadamour.com*

Nemours KidsHealth: *www.kidshealth.org/en/parents*

Positive Parenting Tips: *www.cdc.gov/child-development/positive-parenting-tips*

PositivePsychology: 45 Goal Setting Activities, Exercises, and Games: *www. positivepsychology.com/goal-setting-exercises*

Q.E.D. Foundation: *www.allkindsofminds.org*

Sleep Foundation: Children and Sleep: *www.sleepfoundation.org/children-and-sleep*

Tilt Parenting: *www.tiltparenting.com*

VIA Institute on Character: *www.viacharacter.org*

Podcasts

Ask Lisa: The Psychology of Raising Tweens and Teens with Lisa Damour and Reena Ninan

Full-Tilt Parenting

Power Your Parenting

Raising Good Humans

Index

R

S

About
the Authors

Ellen Braaten, PhD, is Founding Director of the Learning and Emotional Assessment Program at Massachusetts General Hospital and Associate Professor of Psychology at Harvard Medical School. Dr. Braaten is widely recognized as an expert in the field of pediatric neuropsychological and psychological assessment, particularly in the areas of assessing learning disabilities and attentional disorders. She is author or coauthor of many books and articles for parents and professionals.

Hillary Bush, PhD, is a psychologist in private practice in Boston, where she provides neuropsychological assessments and therapy for children, teens, and young adults. Dr. Bush also serves as a part-time faculty member at the University of Massachusetts Boston. She has published articles across many psychology topics for both scientific audiences and the general public.